THE LONG SAFARI

The
Long Safari

BERNARD GLEMSER

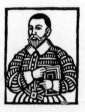

THE BODLEY HEAD
LONDON SYDNEY
TORONTO

Published in the United States of America as
Mr. Burkitt and Africa

Copyright © 1970 by Bernard Glemser
ISBN 0 370 01323 9
Printed in Great Britain for
The Bodley Head Ltd
9 Bow Street, London, WC2E 7AL
by Lowe & Brydone (Printers) Ltd., London
First published in Great Britain 1971

To
V.C.G.

Contents

A*

Introduction

Every now and then something of importance occurs in the scientific world that is more than a scientific event pure and simple, and finds its best expression as a story. Scientific discovery is not entirely a matter of laboratory glassware and sophisticated instruments, of progressing in a series of precise steps from *a* to *b* to *c*. Human beings are involved, and the jump from *a* to *b*, or from *b* to *c*, may be accompanied by spectacular emotional fireworks, by tragedy, comedy, and misunderstandings more appropriate to a novel than a technical paper. One example that comes to mind is *The Double Helix*, by Dr. J. D. Watson, an account of how he and two fellow scientists solved the problem of the structure of DNA, the cellular substance which has been called "the very stuff of life." The discovery, which earned the three men a Nobel Prize, is described in detail in every modern textbook of biology. The *story*, though, is something else. It is full of mischief, uncertainty, decision, indecision; and its central characters are remarkably vivid (who can forget the opening sentence: *I have never seen Francis Crick in a modest mood,* or the mysterious and doomed Rosalind Franklin?).

This book is the story of a series of medical discoveries which began in 1957 and are still continuing. The story's central character is an Irish surgeon, Denis Parsons Burkitt, who early in his life committed himself to work among the people of Africa, and who eventually "happened" to come upon and identify a form of cancer that afflicts many African children. He then set off on a safari of ten thousand miles, with two devoted missionary friends, and literally tracked down the peculiar circumstances in which this tumor occurred. This, though, is only the first part of the story; for Denis Burkitt then went on to discover means for curing the cancer in a significant number of cases.

Whenever any writer announces that he is going to give an account of a cure for a particular form of cancer, the reader should promptly assume an attitude of hard disbelief. Cures for cancer, unfortunately, are exceedingly rare—unless, that is, the cure is accomplished in the conventional manner by means of surgery or radiotherapy. The work of Denis Burkitt and his colleagues, however, has become one of the cornerstones of contemporary cancer research, and it is being followed up by experts all over the world. In a book called *Man Against Cancer* I described Mr. Burkitt's appearance before an audience of cancer specialists (the actual occasion was an address he gave in 1967 at the Sloan-Kettering Institute for Cancer Research in New York): "He has a decided military bearing—the result, perhaps, of his five years of service in the British Army, or of having grown up in Enniskillen, Northern Ireland, which is renowned (he will tell you proudly) as the home of two great regiments. His voice has an Irish lilt, and he cannot resist making a joke or two as he tells about his work in Kampala, Uganda.

"Then the color slides come on the screen. About half are photographs of his African children, with grotesquely distorted faces or swollen bodies, resulting from the tumor which has been given his name. *But each color slide showing a child with a tumor is followed by another color slide showing the same child without a tumor*—cured by a handful of pills or a single injection. The last color slide shows a long line of these children, attired in their bright East African robes, standing in a sunny little street and gazing solemnly at the camera. They are clear-eyed and, as far as any human being can tell, in perfect health." It is not surprising that these photographs invariably bring Mr. Burkitt an ovation.

But an account of the discovery and treatment of a particular form of cancer scarcely sounds like enthralling fireside reading. The reader is herewith assured that it is one of the most remarkable stories in the history of medicine; that it is neither painful nor depressing; and that all the people who participate in the story, without exception, are highly dedicated and highly motivated. Many of the principal characters, indeed, are men of deep religious faith; and although this may be surprising in an age of disbelief and cynicism, it is true to say that if the religious element had been absent the story would have been absent, too. The sequence of discoveries described in this book would not, and probably could not, have occurred, and medical science would have been much poorer in consequence.

A number of scientists helped me most generously in the preparation of this book, and I owe them a profound debt of gratitude. They include Mr. Burkitt himself (who gallantly withstood numerous lengthy and exhausting interviews, and answered a multitude of letters); the Rev. Dr. Hugh C. Trowell; Dr. E. H. Williams; Mr. Peter Clifford; Dr. Dennis H. Wright; Professor M. A. Epstein; Dr. Gilbert Dalldorf; Professor George Klein; Dr. Jan Stjernswärd; Dr. G. B. de Thé; Dr. Malcolm Pike; Dr. Thomas M. Bell; Dr. J. L. Ziegler; Dr. Gertrude Henle and Dr. Werner Henle (in whose laboratories I also had the pleasure of talking to Miss Elaine Hutkin). I am particularly grateful to Professor Sir Ian McAdam for permission to quote from a personal letter; and I am happy indeed to have Mr. Burkitt's permission to print extracts from his diary of the long safari. Several scientists who played an important part in the story were not interviewed, to my great regret, because circumstances prevented our meeting: they include Professor M. S. R. Hutt, Professor J. N. P. Davies, Professor A. J. Haddow, and Dr. C. A. Linsell. I must thank the renowned photographer Fritz Henle for permission to reproduce the portrait of Dr. Werner Henle (his brother) and Dr. Gertrude Henle, as well as the photograph of the charming young scientists who worked on the Burkitt–infectious mononucleosis project, and I am very grateful to the Medical Superintendent of Mulago Hospital, Dr. Y. B. Semambo, for sending me the aerial photograph of the magnificent new hospital buildings. I owe thanks, also, to Dr. Daniel H. Connor, Chief of the Infectious Diseases Branch of the Armed Forces Institute of Pathology in Washington, D.C., for his lively photograph of Denis and Mrs. Burkitt.

Conversations were recorded in New York, Philadelphia, and Grand Rapids; in London, Birmingham, and Salisbury, England; in Nairobi, Kenya; in Kampala, Entebbe, and Arua, Uganda. Once again, the engineer in charge of the recording equipment was my wife, Violetta Constance Glemser.

THE LONG SAFARI

1

View over a Lake

Uganda, at the present time, has only one international airport. It is on the shore of Lake Victoria and it is called Entebbe-Kampala, because it serves both towns.

Kampala, the capital of Uganda, is twenty-one miles away, almost due north, but it is in hilly terrain—the town itself sprawls over seven hills—and jet planes cannot approach it. The airport, therefore, is a few minutes' drive from the center of Entebbe, originally the seat of British government in Uganda and still described as the country's administrative capital. But Uganda is relatively small; its area is about 91,000 square miles, approximately the same as Oregon or Wyoming or the United Kingdom, and it really does not need two capitals. As a result, Entebbe is gradually being divested of its governmental responsibilities, and it now has the appearance of a ghost town. Nothing very much seems to happen from day to day; the atmosphere is relaxed; the pace of life is slow and dreamy.

The main shopping area is unattractive. The shops are

dull, small, crowded, poorly lit. The places to visit are the zoo; the Botanical Gardens, which has a fine stand of rain forest; and—if you have an invitation and are interested in virology— the East African Virus Research Institute. Otherwise there is nothing of great interest. A war memorial, a bank, a post office—nothing wildly exciting.

However, not far from the war memorial is a fine old hotel, the Lake Victoria, where the visitor can while away his time in comfort. It has a swimming pool; there are numerous tables on the lawn, shaded by big umbrellas, where you can enjoy a leisurely afternoon tea; and it is a jumping-off place for safaris to many of the famous game parks—Kagera, Serengeti, Murchison Falls National Park—or to the snowcapped Mountains of the Moon.

Before dinner you can sit on a broad and pleasant balcony drinking waragi, which is distilled from bananas and can be ordered with or without banana flavor. It is the national drink; it is delicious and seems to be nonintoxicating; and it costs only a few pennies.

Below you is an electrical contraption on a tall iron standard, which attracts and kills marauding insects, electrocuting them with a harsh crackle. Beyond, you look across a beautifully manicured golf course; and beyond this, about half a mile away, is the lake. Victoria Nyanza is the second-largest freshwater lake in the world, covering nearly 27,000 square miles (the largest is Lake Superior, covering nearly ·32,000 square miles); it is 250 miles long from north to south, and 150 miles wide, and Scotland would fit into it nicely.

In the evening light it looks exceedingly beautiful. The water is smooth, blue-gray, enticing, and it spreads like an ocean right across the horizon. There are a great many islands on it, with pretty names— Sagitu Island, Lolui Island, Mwama Island, Zinga, Buvu, Lulamba, Serinya, Kalangala,

Bwendero, and countless more. If you arrived here in day-light, flying across the lake from Nairobi, you will have seen many of them from the air, and you must have thought how romantic they look, with their palm trees and unspoiled beaches. It would be wonderful, you may have told yourself, to sail to Dwaji Island or to explore the fabulous Sese Islands. You might even sail to Jinja and discover for yourself the source of the Victoria Nile.

Africa. Enchanted Africa. Mysterious Africa.

But there is something curiously wrong with this picture. Speak to the two friendly and helpful ladies in the hotel travel bureau and they will tell you—most regretfully—that they cannot arrange any excursions for you on Victoria Ny-anza: there is no longer an excursion steamer. And when you go up to the balcony and look out across that enormous expanse of water you will observe that it is almost totally lifeless—at least in terms of human life. Far out, perhaps, there may be a few fishing boats; closer in, at the Entebbe Club, there are a few—very few—small sailboats tied up to moorings.

This is strange. You know that anywhere in Europe, in North America, in Japan, in Australia, a similar expanse of water would be teeming with human beings. There would be sailboats tacking all over the place, and motorboats going much too fast, and water-skiers, and fishermen, and young women splashing each other, because all water sports are joyous and have the power to dispel the dark clouds of the spirit.

Not here. Here man is pointedly absent. There are no dainty sailboats, no noisy motorboats, no children's voices, not even a crying baby. When you become aware of the empti-ness and the silence it is alarming, and baffling. The friendly

ladies in the travel bureau will explain it in a single word:
bilharzia.

Most medical historians spare only a few lines for Theodor
Bilharz. He was a German helminthologist (that is, a scientist who studies worms); he lived from 1825–62; he discovered the tiny worm, or blood fluke, that was named for him
in 1852.

Bilharzia is a parasite, and one of the most dangerous
known to man. It lives its life in a very specific cycle. First,
it is harbored in the fleshy body of a certain kind of freshwater snail. At some stage in its development it leaves the
snail, and for about forty-eight hours it is a free-swimming
tadpole-shaped organism. It may now come in contact with
a human being who is bathing or wading in the water, walking along a wet beach, or sitting in apparent security in a
boat. The organism attaches itself to its new host by means
of suckers, enters through the skin, and is carried to various
organs where it mates, and then proceeds to produce as many
as a thousand eggs a day. Extensive damage is done to the
bladder and the lower part of the colon (some authorities
believe that bilharzia may be responsible for cancer of the
bladder). Meanwhile, great numbers of eggs are passed in
the victim's urine; they hatch, seek out their special freshwater snails, and begin the cycle anew. The disease caused
by bilharzia is known as bilharziasis, or—a term preferred by
many authorities—schistosomiasis.

According to Dr. G. C. Coles, of the Department of
Zoology at Makerere University College, Kampala, bilharzia
infests virtually all the lakes and streams of Uganda. In a
statement printed in the Uganda *Argus* of December 1, 1968,
under a banner headline: WARNING: BILHARZIA IS A KILLER,
Dr. Coles states, "In view of the prevalence of bilharzia and

the fact that in many areas little is known about its distribution, the best advice for people is to avoid all contact with water in rivers, streams, pools and lakes." In the West Nile District alone, it is estimated that 200,000 people have the disease.*

This is only part of the story as it concerns the African continent. All along the Victoria Nile, all along the Albert Nile and the White Nile and the Blue Nile, over a course of 3,500 miles to Cairo and, ultimately, to the great Delta of the Nile discharging into the Mediterranean, the populations are subject to bilharzia infection, and it is the severe organic damage inflicted by the parasite that debilitates these people. They are literally drained of energy, and thus incapable of doing the work that would lead them out of poverty. The development of irrigation programs, indispensable to an expanding economy, only brings bilharzia closer to more and more human beings.

The obvious solution is to eliminate the freshwater snails, which are essential to the life cycle of bilharzia. Unfortunately, even if this were feasible (in some African nations the cost would be more than the total national income) it might disturb the entire ecology of tropical and North Africa. All that can be done is to provide treatment for people suffering from the disease; but again, any full-scale treatment for the millions of men, women, and children at present infected is far beyond the resources of the available medical services.

And bilharzia is only one of Africa's health problems.

* The well-known zoologist, explorer, and television personality Jack Paar reports seeing a sign on the banks of a lake in Uganda: WARNING: SWIMMING IN THIS LAKE IS SUICIDE.

The light on majestic Victoria Nyanza is a little less bright now; and this is the time of day when the mosquitoes become active, dancing in their trillions on the fringes of the lake. But you have no need to worry unduly about them. You have been taking your anti-malaria pills regularly, and before you flew here you had all the requisite inoculations: smallpox, yellow fever, typhoid, paratyphoid, cholera, tetanus, and perhaps polio. You are, indeed, in far better shape to resist infection than most of the Africans who live here. Not many of them have ever had an inoculation of any kind.

It is a curious fact that the African is now almost totally secure from attack by the wild and savage animals that are supposed to surround him. Few Africans today, even those living in the bush, see a lion from one year to the next; and very few—adults or children—go to make a lion's dinner. Any sensible leopard stays as far from man (Man the Coatmaker) as possible; the threat from rampaging elephants is not excessively high; crocodiles in most areas are, by and large, a tourist attraction, although one would be rash to tempt them; snakes are troublesome but by no means as severe a menace as they are in India.

One of the major threats to the African, unfortunately, comes from physical violence: heads are bashed in, throats are slit, poison is slipped into the family beer. Broken bones, knife wounds, infected bites (*human* bites), fill the emergency wards of every African hospital.

But by far the greatest threat arises from forms of life the African never sees: viruses, bacteria, protozoa, in a tremendous variety of forms, causing a staggering variety of illnesses.

To list thèm all would be depressing in the extreme. Naming just a few will be sufficient to give some idea of the fearful burden of disease carried by the African people, sapping their vitality and thwarting their progress.

First and foremost is malaria—massive, inescapable malaria. In tropical Africa this is primarily a disease of children, who are subject to repeated infection almost from birth. If the child survives, and passes through adolescence, some sort of immunity or resistance to malaria often develops.

There is amebic dysentery, also a deadly disease of childhood. Bilharziasis is also common among children. There are yaws, and hookworm, and filariasis (which, among other things, causes elephantiasis). There is trypanosomiasis, or sleeping sickness, spread by the tsetse fly. There is onchocerciasis,* another parasitic infection, spread by the bite of the black fly, which may cause blindness and complete or partial deafness: vast areas of Africa have been abandoned by man because of this pestilence, after the people have endured mass blindness for generations. There is leishmaniasis, or kala-azar, or dumdum fever, yet another parasitic infection, transmitted by sandflies. There are tuberculosis, venereal disease, leprosy, smallpox, yellow fever. There are numerous kinds of fungus infection, some extremely serious.

The total outcome is grim. In most African nations, half of all the children die before they reach the age of five. At the other end of the scale, you see very few Africans, male or female, with white hair, for only 10 percent live beyond the age of forty. In general, the African does not live long enough to succumb to heart disease or cancer, the leading causes of death in Western man, and the reason is that, for the most

* This is usually pronounced *onco-ser-sý-asis.* "Onchocerca" means barbed tail and refers to the parasite's method of attaching itself to its victim; "asis," like "osis," simply means a medical condition or state.

part, heart disease and cancer make their appearance in the fifth and sixth decades of the life span. There are exceptions to this generalization (some forms of cancer are prevalent in certain parts of Africa, rare in the West); but on the whole it is the communicable diseases that menace and encircle the African, those diseases that are firmly established in his environment, that thrive in tropical heat and humidity and in the conditions of poverty.

Disease, then, is the major problem of the mass of human beings in Uganda, and Kenya, and every other African nation. The Ugandan government spends one-tenth of the national income on health services—the World Bank, which has a say in such matters, will not approve spending more—and this is simply not enough to pay for the medical resources to cope with the situation.

In these circumstances it is remarkable that a disease now called Burkitt's lymphoma, accounting for only a few hundred lives a year (not in any single country but over a large part of tropical Africa) should have attracted the interest of scientists all over the world. "In the total context of disease in Africa," Mr. Burkitt once observed, "it is only an infinitesimal fleabite." But a fleabite of a special kind, and of special importance.

2

Forerunners

The outside world has responded to the African's particular vulnerability in many different ways throughout the centuries: slavery, colonialism, exploitation, pillage, murder. There has also been—and it deserves to be remembered—another kind of response: compassion, a form of giving, as against the many forms of taking.

This is an age that regards with suspicion the motives of any white man who went to Africa uninvited, and many people dismiss (or condemn) the early missionaries as fanatics who served to open the way for all the evils of imperialism, who kept the African in subjugation by threatening him with eternal hellfire while the traders and colonists stripped the continent of its wealth. The picture is untrue, and we do these men a profound injustice if we judge them in such distorted terms.

Two of the early African missionaries have a place in this book. Their influence is indirect, but it is nevertheless vital. The first, of course, is David Livingstone, a man of incredible

resolution and spiritual force. He has perplexed all his biogra-
phers; in some respects he is completely incomprehensible to
modern readers; yet, as you follow him year by year, his
accomplishments, his mistakes, his failures, his strength, fill
you with awe. He is elemental.

Most of us have forgotten what poverty and hardship
really mean, and it is worth recalling how men made their
way in the world a century and a half ago. Livingstone was
born in Blantyre, Scotland, in 1813. At the age of ten he was
put to work in a cotton factory. Out of his first week's wages
he bought a Latin grammar, and somehow or other he mem-
orized it sentence by sentence as he tended the spinning
jennies. His workday was from six o'clock in the morning until eight at night; when he finished he hurried on to evening
classes, which lasted until ten o'clock, and when he arrived
home—a single room served for the entire family: father,
mother, and four other children—he continued to read until
midnight. He was at last prepared to enter college in Glas-
gow when he was twenty-three, and began studies in chemistry, medicine, Greek, and divinity. There, he wrote later,
"in the glow of love which Christianity inspires, I soon resolved to devote my life to the alleviation of human misery;
and therefore set myself to obtain a medical education in
order to be qualified for that enterprise." He completed his
medical studies in London and was accepted (not altogether
with enthusiasm) by the London Missionary Society. His
hope was to be sent to China. The Directors of the Society
intended to send him to the West Indies. Eventually it was
agreed that he should go to Africa.

He went out as a missionary doctor, but fairly soon his
attitude hardened. In a letter to one of his tutors, the Rev.
Richard Cecil, he wrote: "I did not at first intend to give up
all attention to medicine and the treatment of disease, but

now I feel it my duty to have as little to do with it as possible. I shall attend to none but severe cases in future, and my reasons for this determination are I think good. The spiritual amelioration of the people is the object for which I came, but I cannot expect God to advance this by my instrumentality if much of my time is spent in mere temporal amelioration." He believed fervently that the immortal souls of those who had not accepted the Christian gospel would perish in the Great Assize—the Last Judgment; thus the saving of souls became his primary purpose. It was then that he began his travels in southern Africa, pressing north into what he called —and what was in fact—the dark interior: territory which had not been explored by any Europeans, where Christianity was totally unknown. "It was the dream of the imperialist Cecil Rhodes, a generation later," writes Dr. George Seaver in his biography of Livingstone, "that the uncolonized portion of the map of South Africa, from the Cape to the Zambesi, should be painted red for Britain. It was the dream of the missionary David Livingstone that the whole continent should be painted white for Christ."

His journeys extended from the Cape northward, deep into the Congo and almost to the equator; and from Quelimane on the Indian Ocean right across Africa to Luanda on the Atlantic Ocean. It is estimated that he explored one-third of the continent, at a time when it was largely a blank space on the map, and he filled in the geographical details with extraordinary accuracy. Ultimately, the urge to explore unknown Africa, to press on and on, overshadowed the missionary impulse; but his greatest passion, inflamed by the atrocities of the Portuguese and Arab slavers, was to put an end to the slave trade. "The sights I have seen, though common incidents of the (slave) traffic, are so nauseous that I always strive to drive them from memory. . . . The slaving scenes come back unbidden, and make me start up at dead of night, horrified by their vividness." And in a letter to the *New York Herald*, asking for aid to end the traffic in slaves, he concluded, "All I can say in my solitude is, may Heaven's rich blessing come down on everyone—American, English, Turk—who will help to heal this Open Sore of the World." The words are engraved on his tomb in Westminster Abbey.

The effect of Livingstone upon the young men and women of his time is indescribable. Sixteen years after he first went to Africa he returned home for a visit. He spent six months writing his great *Missionary Travels,* a book of nearly 700 pages, which instantly ran through nine printings; and he then toured the country, giving talks to large audiences, receiving acclamation everywhere. Dr. Seaver writes: "He was on the crest of a tremendous wave of public enthusiasm which happily coincided with a wave of national prosperity. He was already an established hero. In the eyes of his countrymen nothing comparable with his achievements had occurred since Drake sailed round the world. His sudden disclosure of the resources, both human and material . . . was spectacular, and henceforth Central Africa became a focus of national interest—political, mercantile, and missionary."

Livingstone's message to those who cheered his accomplishments was fierce and direct: "Do you carry on the work which I have begun. I leave it with you." Nothing more needed to be said.

The last journeys of Livingstone ended in tragedy. He died in 1873, after fearful hardships, searching—mistakenly—for the four mysterious fountains which he believed might be the source of the Nile. Henry Morton Stanley, who had found him virtually dying two years earlier at Ujiji on Lake Tanganyika, set himself to carry on Livingstone's work. He marched into Africa with a small army of followers, reached Lake Victoria, made his way up the eastern side of the lake, survived encounters with hostile tribesmen (and hippos); and in due course met Mutesa, ruler of the largest kingdom of Uganda. (The name of the country is Uganda; the name of this ancient kingdom is Buganda; the name of a native of Buganda is Muganda, and the plural is Baganda; anything relating to Buganda is Kiganda; the name of the language is Luganda.)

A famous dispatch from Stanley, printed in the London *Daily Telegraph* in November 1875, testifies to his powers of persuasion. It reads, in part: "I have indeed undermined Islamism so much here that Mutesa is determined henceforth, until he is better informed, to observe the Christian Sabbath as well as the Moslem Sabbath, and the great captains have unanimously consented to this. . . .

"But oh, that some pious, practical missionary would come here! What a field and harvest ripe for the sickle of civilization. Mutesa would give him anything he desired—houses, land, cattle, ivory, etc.; he might call a province his own one day. It is not the mere teacher that is wanted here. The Bishops of Great Britain collected, with the classic youth of Oxford and Cambridge, would affect nothing by mere talk with the intelligent folk of Uganda. It is the practical Christian tutor who can teach people how to become Christians, cure their diseases, construct dwellings, understand and exemplify agriculture and turn his hand to anything, like a sailor—this is the man who is wanted. Such a man if he could be found, would become the Saviour of Africa. He must be tied to no one church or sect, but profess God and His Son and the moral law, and live a blameless Christian, inspired by liberal principles and charity to all men, and devout faith in Heaven. He must belong to no one nation in particular, but the entire white race. Such a man Mutesa, King of Uganda, Usoga, Unyoro and Karagwe—a kingdom three hundred and sixty geographical miles in length by fifty in breadth—invites to repair to him. He has begged me to tell the white men that if they will only come to him he will give them all they want. Nowhere is there in all the Pagan world a more promising field for a mission than Uganda. . . .

"Here, gentlemen, is your opportunity—embrace it! The people on the shores of the Nyanza call upon you!"

Within a few weeks, £24,000 ($120,000, an immense sum in 1875) had been subscribed for a mission to the court of Mutesa, and volunteers began to hurry out to embrace the opportunity. They found to their bewilderment that Stanley had allowed himself to be hypnotized by his own eloquence. The welcome they had been promised was not forthcoming. They were constantly harassed, a number of them were brutally murdered, many were killed in the civil wars that seemed to go on endlessly in Central Africa; and many, inevitably, died of disease. The result, of course, was that the missionary fervor only increased.

In November 1896, twelve missionaries sent out by the Church Missionary Society began a safari from Mombasa, on the east coast, to Kampala. One of the men in the party was Albert Ruskin Cook, a young doctor; there were two women, one of them Miss Katherine Timpson, whom Cook later married.

The journey took eighty-four days. The twelve missionaries marched more than 700 miles, through forests, swamps, desert, and over mountains. Wild animals were a serious threat. In many places the natives were openly hostile. The white men and women came down with dysentery, a terrible affliction in such primitive conditions; the carriers came down with the usual tropical diseases.

On the very first day that the party entered Uganda, at Ngogwe, halfway between Jinja and Kampala, Dr. Cook treated 226 patients.

It was only a foretaste of what awaited him. Unlike Livingstone, Cook's purpose in coming to Africa was to organize a medical mission and hospital. His concern was to heal the bodies of the Africans, as a first step toward saving their immortal souls; and he set to work in a shed with a mud floor, transforming it into a serviceable hospital in which he could see patients and perform operations, with Katherine as his nurse to administer anesthetics and apply dressings. Soon a larger hospital was built, consisting of two huts, each with six beds. Later he moved to a more ambitious hospital with fifty beds, described as "the finest building in Uganda, shaped like a double Greek cross, 120 feet long and 40 feet across at the widest part."

Livingstone, crying out passionately about the Open Sore of the World, was referring to the vicious slave traffic in Central Africa; but the term could be applied literally to the great lake and the territory surrounding it. Before the arrival of Albert and Katherine Cook there were no medical facilities at all in the whole of Uganda, except an ineffectual mission dispensary. The healers of the sick were the witch doctors or muttering old sorceresses. The average man (Rousseau's "noble savage") was generally in a wretched state of health, riddled with disease, weakened by malnutrition, ignorant, and oppressed by murderous tyrants whose forces of law and order consisted of regiments of executioners. The average man's wife had her first pregnancy at the age of about twelve, was exhausted by successive pregnancies until she was in her early twenties, and then literally withered away into premature old age.

Dr. Cook's little hospital was besieged by patients every day. That was not enough for him. First on foot, later on the first bicycle seen in Uganda, he went to tend the sick in outlying villages, and the people gathered in crowds to be examined and receive medication. *Everybody* seemed to be sick. On one trip, accompanied by the irresistible Katherine, he tended more than five thousand patients and performed fifty major operations. On another occasion he set out for a district where smallpox was raging and inoculated three thousand people—more than eight hundred in a single day.

This was a man truly devoted to the noble practice of medicine. His duty was to heal the sick, and he did all that was possible in utterly primitive conditions. Many of the tropical diseases were not yet understood by medical scientists; and early in his career, for example, Dr. Cook was forced to look on helplessly as an epidemic of sleeping sickness killed more than a quarter of a million Baganda. In 1916, during World War I, the Cooks and a few trained doctors, helped by some medical assistants, had to deal with the simultaneous outbreak of four epidemics: smallpox, cerebrospinal meningitis, choleraic dysentery, and—most serious of all—bubonic plague.

Gradually the truth became clear: the Baganda people were facing extinction. Statistics for a seven-year period, from 1914 to 1920, showed only 68,000 births, against 97,000 deaths and 7,000 stillbirths. Infant mortality was appallingly high: Jack Cook, Albert's brother, found that 70 percent of infants died before they were a week old. In one district, births for that seven-year period were 16,000, while deaths— including stillbirths—totalled 31,000. Albert and Katherine Cook, by establishing hospital services, by training African medical assistants and midwives, by persuading the government to take action against venereal disease, by encouraging education programs, may well have saved the Bagandan nation.

Cook's biographer, Brian O'Brien,* describes him as he was seen by a contemporary: "A quiet, yet stubborn man, medium height, chunky and quick moving. Red beard, mild blue eyes, and a very nice sense of humor. . . . He had a nerve of iron; he'd take risks that would make your blood run cold. When he was called, he set off, no matter where; through elephant country with no protection whatever, down the lake in a canoe that leaked like a basket or through neck-deep swamps that crawled with snakes. He was absolutely without fear. He believed that God had sent him to do a job and his logical scientific mind made it impossible to think God would let anything interfere with that job."

The passion with which Albert and Katherine Cook did their work (on the allowance given to married missionaries of £15—$75—a month) inevitably undermined their health. They were worn down, writes O'Brien, by the long journeys, the crowds of patients, drenching rains, the night chills of the mountains and the sweltering heat of the swamps. "They both suffered recurring bouts of malaria. Katherine frequently collapsed with blinding headaches, and insomnia made her nights a dread. The doctor's leg, swollen to twice its normal size by phlebitis (the result of typhoid contracted from a patient) tormented him incessantly; chronic dysentery, held in check by morphine, drained his strength." In

* *That Good Physician: The Life and Work of Albert and Katherine Cook of Uganda.* London: Hodder and Stoughton, 1962.

B

1938, Katherine died of encephalitis, after a severe attack of malaria. Albert Cook lived until 1951, loved and respected by the people of Uganda. He had been knighted some twenty years earlier, thus joining the small, distinguished group of missionary knights; but at his death he received an even more signal honor. Watched by grieving crowds, his coffin was carried by the great chiefs of Buganda to the cathedral on Namirembe Hill; and there, in a grave lined with royal bark cloth, he was buried beside his dear Katherine. It was the only royal funeral ever accorded to a white man in Uganda.

It is unlikely that he felt he had done anything unusual or remarkable. After Cook's death an African wrote: "The arrival of Sir Albert Cook fifty years ago was the greatest event as far as the progress of my country was concerned." But for Albert Cook himself the key to all his conduct was doing, as well as he could, the work that had been mapped out for him. Only a fool would argue that he was mistaken in his beliefs.

After a particularly arduous safari, treating patients who were suffering from sleeping sickness, leprosy, blackwater fever, hydrocele—the whole gamut of tropical disease—he wrote in his journal: "Is it any wonder that we magnify our office, and that we love this happy work with an ever growing affection; and conversely, is it not amazing that from our overstocked profession at home, so few—pitifully few, considering the respective needs—Christian doctors come out?" It is reminiscent of Livingstone's challenge, *Do you carry on the work which I have begun. I leave it with you.* And, as with Livingstone, Cook's message did not go unheeded.

3

Making of a Surgeon

Denis Parsons Burkitt was born in February 1911, in Enniskillen, Northern Ireland, the county town of Co. Fermanagh. It lies on Lough Erne, not very far from Donegal Bay, which opens onto the Atlantic Ocean; and it has the distinction of being the only town in the world to have two regiments named after it. The population is about eight thousand.

The Burkitt family traces its ancestry to the Norman invasion of Ireland. Midway in the family history, one of its members married a daughter of Oliver Cromwell (who is considered by many Irishmen to be a monster of satanic proportions). A certain independence of mind is also evident in Denis Burkitt's maternal forebears. His mother came from County Cork; *her* father, an architect who designed the handsome Cork courthouse, was offered a knighthood by the British government and turned it down, declaring that he preferred to live and die as plain Mr. Hill and wanted nothing else.

21

James Parsons Burkitt, father of Denis, was one of seven children. *His* father, also a man of independent spirit, was a Presbyterian minister in a totally Catholic environment in the west of Ireland, and it is not surprising that he lived in considerable poverty. No doubt as a result of their upbringing, each of his five sons did remarkably well. One went to India in the Civil Service and became a Resident, corresponding to Governor of a State. One went to Guatemala and did valuable work on ancient monuments. Another became Senior Engineer in the Punjab, and was later associated with the Aswan Dam project, for which he was decorated by the British government.

Another of the five sons, Roland Wilks Burkitt, went out to Nairobi in 1911 when, according to his biographer, "it was but a wood-and-iron dorp scattered over the plains."* He was highly qualified, being a Fellow of the Royal College of Surgeons of Ireland, and for many years he was the town's only private practitioner.

"A very remarkable man was my Uncle Roland," Denis Burkitt once said of him, obviously with great pride: "He was an eccentric man, but people who stand for something very specific in rather perverse society are bound to be considered eccentric if they have a centre different from the society in which they live. He was a man of the *utmost* standard of morals: if he thought the Governor (of Kenya) had done anything wrong he would tell him so instantly." And again: "My Uncle Roland was an absolutely fearless man for what was right. He was a tremendous student of Scripture, but rather *anti* the established church. He started a little Sunday

* *Under The Sun: A Memoir of Dr. R. W. Burkitt, of Kenya,* by J. R. Gregory. 119 pages. This was privately printed in Kenya and is undated.

meeting in Nairobi, which in a different form still goes on today, fifty years later."

Roland Burkitt was clearly larger than life. He might have sprung fully armed from one of the novels of Joyce Cary: a blunt and vigorous man, supremely confident in himself and with little patience for the rest of the world. Some of the methods of treatment he introduced were new, and he applied them so thoroughly and ruthlessly that among the settlers of Nairobi he was known as "Kill or Cure Burkitt." He believed, for instance, that cold packs—or better still, cold baths—were helpful in treating patients with high fever. "During the influenza epidemics and in the malarial seasons," writes his biographer, Dr. Gregory, "Burkitt had patients all over the town in cold baths, under wet sheets, being sprayed with watering cans or merely being sponged. . . . Woe betide the relative or nurse who abandoned treatment before the desired result was achieved, but some people were not above setting an African servant on watch to give warning of the doctor's approach, so that a comfortable bed could be abandoned for the bathroom. Prominent and worthy citizens, in response to a warning from the watcher, could be seen rushing in their pelts along passages to the bathroom and plunging into a cold bath, while the doctor's Ford car chugged up to the house. . . . If a thought struck him in the middle of the night that some point had been overlooked or some other line of treatment was desirable, he would not hesitate to get up and drive off to his patient, arousing the whole household to achieve his object. A very sick patient could be quite certain that Burkitt would arrive to see him between five and six in the morning."

One of the best tales illustrating his belief in cold treatment for fever concerns a very big woman living some distance out in the country. "He found her with a very high temperature," Dr. Gregory writes. "He decided to bring her into hospital in Nairobi. Her relatives wanted to wrap her in blankets, afraid she would get cold, but Burkitt refused. Instead, he insisted that she should travel naked in the back of his open Ford car. On the way in, he stopped and took her temperature. He found it was dropping, so he took off his coat and wrapped it around her. As the story goes, the patient eventually reached the hospital dressed in all of Burkitt's clothes, while he arrived naked. When I plied him with this story, a twinkle came into his eye as he said, 'Ah, Gregory! People are apt to exaggerate.' "

What few of his patients knew was that he had a passion for his work: "New methods would be studied until he had mastered the minutest detail. He would come away (from visits to London) after weeks of watching the leading surgeons, satisfied and delighted if he had learned one new "tip," and what he knew was at the disposal of all those who wished to learn. His generosity in this respect knew no bounds."

But he had very fixed ideas, says Gregory, on how women should dress and behave: "He considered that women should wear long dresses. When it became fashionable for women to don frocks that stopped above the knees, he inaugurated a preaching campaign against them. He would look at a woman's knees in a fixed way and cause her much embarrassment by saying, 'A woman's knees are very ugly. You should cover them up.' . . . Mrs. Burkitt was a particularly beautiful woman, tall, slender, graceful and well featured. . . . She met what she considered to be an impossible situation by having her dresses fitted with two belts, one of which enabled her to wear them long to please her husband, and one which held them up to the fashionable length to please the dictates of fashion. It caused immense amusement to her friends to see her skirt being lengthened the moment Dr. Burkitt appeared on the scene."

On the other hand, he was a man to be trusted. "He would put everything else aside to go where he thought he was most needed. In those days calls came from great distances over two or three hundred miles away, and in wet weather, over bad roads, they could be nightmare journeys. Every detail for getting his car through swampy patches had to be dealt with, and medical equipment to meet all emergencies had to be taken. . . . On occasion he travelled into the Northern Frontier of Kenya, which in those days was a five days' journey, to bring in a hunter who had met with an accident and had fractured a thigh. He travelled hundreds of miles into Tanganyika Territory at the request of his colleagues to see desperately ill patients and, if necessary, he would transport them back to Nairobi in his car, spending days on the journey."

Eccentric? Perhaps so. But one would like to see a little more of this eccentricity in contemporary medical practice.

James Burkitt, the second in age of the five sons, was the only one to stay home. He became county surveyor in Fermanagh and was responsible for all the county roads and for the building of several bridges. He had a "little hobby" (according to his son Denis) which none of the family took seriously: birdwatching. Now, birdwatching is a hobby that few non-birdwatchers are inclined to take seriously; furthermore, James Burkitt chose to study, in particular, the robins in his ten-acre garden—the sprightly, lovable little robin redbreast who for countless years has appeared on Christmas cards as a symbol of good cheer and good will toward all men—and nobody could take *that* very seriously. But James Burkitt became the world authority on robins. He was the first naturalist to band birds so that their individual behavior could be studied and recorded; and, consequently, he was able to plot for the first time the territory inhabited—and so jealously guarded—by each bird. He showed that far from being happy, good-natured little creatures, male robins are pugnacious bullies. Each robin was allotted a number; its location in the garden was marked on a map; its movements were followed minutely; and its history was recorded on long foolscap pages, written in an unusually fine Italian hand. The great ornithologist David Lack named him as one of the seven men who have contributed most to the understanding of bird behavior (among the other six were Edmund Selous and Julian Huxley), a distinction that came as a surprise to his family, which had never realized he was such an authority.

He, too, was a man of deep Christian faith; and this—unlike birdwatching—he successfully imparted to his children. Perhaps something of the birdwatching habit was also imparted; in another form it may have played an important part in Denis Burkitt's later development, leading him to become a careful and astute observer and a patient keeper of records. Denis has acknowledged this influence in a typical manner: "I feel very much that anything one has accomplished is due to what one has received, in two senses. First of all, at birth, through inheritance from both parents. Secondly, what one receives through life." The point is made in a text from Corinthians, framed and hanging on the wall of his London office: *What do you possess that was not given you? If then you really received it as a gift why take the credit to yourself?* In the Authorized King James Version the text reads: *For who maketh thee to differ from another? and what hast thou that thou didst not receive? Now if thou didst receive it why dost thou glory, as if thou hadst not re-*

ceived it? It is a simple argument that blunts the edge of conceit.

At school (as he recalls it now) Denis Burkitt was poor to mediocre at everything except mathematics. An undistinguished child, according to his own account.

When he was eleven years old he suffered an accident which had severe effects later on: "Several boys were throwing stones. One of the stones hit me in the eye."

He wore glasses at the time. The glasses were broken, and he lost his right eye. There were no immediate psychological results—the accident worried his parents more than it worried him. He was in a hospital for five weeks, and he remembers most vividly the great joy of being presented with a steam engine as compensation, *a real, working steam engine,* something to delight any boy. And eventually he received a fine blue matching glass eye, so perfectly made that few people recognize it for what it is.

Upon his release from the hospital, his mother sent him and his brother Robin (eighteen months younger than Denis) to a preparatory school in Anglesey, North Wales. Three years later the boys went on to Cheltenham, and four years later they were admitted to the University of Dublin.

At this point certain elements not commonly found in accounts of contemporary medical science become more and more important. Relatively few scientists today are willing to ascribe their achievements to Divine Guidance, or Divine Will, or Divine Plan. Here there is a fundamental and vitally important difference: the principal character in this narrative, and some others who appear later, are convinced of the immanence of God; they have complete faith in His guidance, complete trust in His goodness, absolute reliance that He

B*

will heed their prayers and that His word will be made clear to them; and their conduct in all things is rooted in the Christian ethic. For the reader with similar religious beliefs no further explanation is necessary. For the reader without any deep religious beliefs no further explanation is possible. But whichever way he leans, it will be an interesting exercise for the reader to test his beliefs or nonbeliefs against what occurs in the story from now on.

Denis Burkitt was eighteen years old when he went to Dublin University, and he and his brother were firmly—passionately—committed to one idea: they would do anything, anything in the world, except become doctors. Robin, therefore, started to study modern languages; Denis, therefore, started to study engineering; and both ended as surgeons.

Engineering was enjoyable enough, but it aroused no great enthusiasm in Denis's heart or mind. He did not excel in it, he found his first year colorless, and he made few friends. But the change to medicine did not come about as a result of consultations with any secular advisers: "I attribute it to a spiritual committal to follow what was God's will for me. . . . I made it very much a matter of prayer, and the more I prayed about it the more I felt an overwhelming conviction that God was calling me to make this change. It was made clear to me that medicine was what I was meant to be doing. I had no doubts about it at all. For a time I found it difficult to pluck up the courage to switch over my career, but I felt I must do it. I had asked for guidance, and if I turned back and took what seemed to be an easier way I would always blame myself."

He was now set for two years of pre-clinical studies, and then three years of clinical work. With a foundation of spiritual assurance and a new sense of direction, he moved up from being a mediocre engineer to third or fourth from the top in his medical courses. He was wholly gripped by medicine—"thrilled by it," he says, "thrilled all the way through."

Now, also, he met the people who were to prove—after his family—the greatest formative influence in his life: a group of men at the university who had a faith that governed completely their behavior, their motives, and their thought.

This group originated with three men who returned to study medicine at Dublin University after the First World War and who, in Denis Burkitt's words, "had come into a personal experience of what faith in Christ could mean in their lives." One was Patrick Kerr Dixon, who eventually went out to found a hospital in the Congo and died there; the second was C. P. Martin, who eventually went to McGill University as Professor of Anatomy; the third was David Torrens, who remained in Dublin and became Professor of Physiology and Dean of the Medical School.

These men did not arise, so to speak, as a result of spontaneous spiritual generation. They were inspired by a still larger and more influential group which had its beginnings in Cambridge at the end of the last century, when a very strong movement of dedicated Christians was centered around seven men who were either Blues* or noted scholars and who went out to serve as missionaries in China. The powerful influence of the Cambridge Seven spread to other universities in Britain, resulting in the Intervarsity Christian Fellowship which, in turn, has had a far-reaching international impact. In later years Denis Burkitt was to meet members of these groups wherever he traveled; and the common

---

* Blues are athletes who have won the distinction of wearing their university color: light blue for Cambridge, dark blue for Oxford.

bond, the shared faith and understanding, were of enormous value.

The changeover from engineering to medicine occurred in 1930, when Denis was nineteen years old; and it is interesting, for the sake of perspective, to look back on the scene as it was then. The economic crisis leading to the Great Depression had already occurred in the United States, with grim repercussions all over the world. A couple of years earlier the first Five-Year Plan had been inaugurated in Russia; in many countries—Germany and France, particularly—the international communist movement, encouraged by the widespread economic distress, seemed to be gathering sufficient strength to challenge the shaky capitalist system. Writers such as George Bernard Shaw and H. G. Wells, who offered a sort of utopian socialism as a cure for the world's ills and at the same time advocated rebellion against middle-class morality, had profoundly affected the minds of large numbers of young men and women troubled by the breakdown of established values. Sigmund Freud and D. H. Lawrence, following other paths through the wilderness, offered solutions that seemed on the whole merely to add new problems to the old ones.

Denis Burkitt's path at that time was over a different mountain. "In those days," he comments, "I was much more narrow in my faith than I am today. Youth is always rather intolerant. I never went to the theatre, I hardly ever went to the cinema, I did not dance. And yet I can see that there was a value to it, because we channeled ourselves, we steered away from the groups who accepted everything. To some extent, in life only what is narrow is forceful and effective. A river that becomes wider and wider is likely to turn into a swamp, whereas a narrow river has force and power and direction. And I think that people often use the word *narrow* in a derogatory sense when they apply it to religious beliefs, but no athlete is going to get to the Olympic Games unless he stays in strict training and no scholar is going to get to the top unless he stays clear of time-wasting dissipation."

The Dublin group held meetings once a week; speakers came to address the group; friends outside the group were invited "to be helped in the same way that we had been helped." Members of the group met to confirm and enlarge their experience, to help each other, and there was always a clear understanding between these men that if they were to be of any real value in the world they must go out to the man in need. But, Burkitt insists, everything ultimately is based on the personal dealings between a man and God: "I have always in my life put more emphasis on personal daily devotion than outward church attendance—on a daily search for communion with God. I learned this in college, with my college friends, and I've kept it up ever since. Every morning, even now, when my wife and I get up we make ourselves our morning tea, and I bring morning tea to the family; and we then have half an hour or so just sitting up in bed, for prayer, for thought, for Bible reading, and so on. It gives me time to get orientated, and I've found it of immense value."

At the end of five years he passed out second in his class. There were two jobs as house surgeons available at his teaching hospital and he would have been glad to accept one of them in order to stay in Dublin; but one went to the man who was top of the class, the other to a man who had been captain of the football team and who had played for Ireland and who, in his own special way, could be said to have done much for the hospital.

Ireland could not offer an abundance of jobs and Burkitt,

like most of his class, went to various house jobs in England.
A curious period followed. He went to Chester, in the west
of England, as house surgeon for six months, then back for
six months to his teaching hospital in Dublin. Then he shot
up north to Preston, in Lancashire, where to widen his experience he "did" eyes, as well as ear, nose, and throat surgery. Then, feeling the need for higher qualifications, he went
down to Poole, in Dorset, as Senior Resident Officer, a position somewhat senior to house surgeon. Then, having saved
some money, he left hospital work for six months and went
up to Edinburgh, where with one of his best and oldest
friends, Guy Timmis, he found lodgings with full board at
two guineas a week (about ten and a half dollars, a sum that
he and Timmis considered to be scandalously exorbitant, if
not downright extravagant).

In due course the two men took the examination for Fellow of the Royal College of Surgeons. "I passed," he says,
"and Guy failed. It should have been the other way about."
But now he could put the magic letters F.R.C.S.E. after his
name (the *E* standing for Edinburgh); and from now on he
was entitled to be addressed—as surgeons in Britain are tradi-
tionally addressed—as Mr. Burkitt. For Dr. Timmis there
were few regrets. He went out to Africa in the government
service, and today he runs a leper colony in Tanzania.

4

Mr. Burkitt Goes to Sea

Young Mr. Burkitt—the year was 1938 and he was no more than twenty-seven years old—had now reached a turning point in his life. He had his F.R.C.S.E. in his pocket. The question was, what should he do with it, what use should he make of it? The Royal College of Surgeons does not hand out its Fellowships lightly or indiscriminately. You may have superlative medical talents, you may be a great healer, but that is far from enough. The Fellowship is awarded to a man only when the Royal College of Surgeons is fully satisfied that he meets its standards as a surgeon, and for no other reason.

Thus, acquiring his Fellowship meant, among other things, that his market value had gone up substantially. He could quite reasonably look forward to better and more lucrative appointments. Given a few years to establish himself, he could anticipate a comfortable income, a comfortable life. Successful surgeons are the maharajahs of medicine. They are the darlings of the income tax collector, they are revered by the people who sell Rolls-Royce limousines. And, of course, if a surgeon is good, if he knows his job thoroughly, if he can go inside the human body with confidence and take care of a perilous situation, he deserves every penny of his fee. It is better for the patient to give up his bank balance than to give up the ghost.

But Burkitt was still powerfully influenced by his college friends, by the special nature of his college experiences. There was a vast need among less fortunate people overseas for precisely those services he was fitted to offer, and he knew it too well. The call was strong. It had not yet crystallized, it was not yet specific, but it pressed upon him and he was not sure what to do about it. He needed time to think and time to pray. And finally, in typically Burkitt fashion, he signed as ship's surgeon on a cargo ship, the *Glen Shiel* of the Blue Funnel Line, and he sailed off to Manchuria.

The voyage, out and back, lasted five months. No more than twelve passengers may be carried on a cargo ship, but most of the time the *Glen Shiel* carried none at all. The crew was Chinese, and Burkitt had little to do in his official capacity beyond pulling a few teeth. There was a minimum of social activities, and he was left alone to think, to read, to seek some solution to his problem.

In certain respects it was precisely what a great many other young men were doing in those troubled years. Few of them had Denis Burkitt's qualifications. They signed up on cargo ships as deck hands, as anything, in order to get away and think, and seek adventure, and find a meaningful way to live. Young men today have the same urge: for some reason they have difficulty thinking at home, they are convinced that they will think more clearly five thousand miles away. Today, though, things have changed; the maritime unions are not particularly sympathetic toward young men who want to work their passage to foreign parts for the purpose of thinking, and something rather valuable has been lost.

The trip to Manchuria remains vividly in Burkitt's memory. The *Glen Shiel* sailed through the Mediterranean to Haifa; then to Port Said and through the Suez Canal to Port Taufiq; across the Arabian Sea to Colombo; then to Penang and Singapore; up the South China Sea to Hong Kong, and on to Shanghai and Dairen.

When he returned his mind was firmly made up about one thing: it would be impossible for him to join what he called "the surgical rat race" at home. He was one step nearer his ultimate destination.

The details of his future commitment still remained to be worked out in his mind. Meanwhile, he had a living to earn, and he went to Plymouth as Resident Surgical Officer.

Here two things happened which he could not possibly have anticipated. The first was the outbreak of World War II, which caused him considerable anxiety—he was unable to decide what to do, whether to leave Plymouth or stay on for another six months after completing his first tour of duty. "And again, as my custom was, I prayed about it; and again, as has happened to me in certain critical times in my life, a verse of Scripture stood out and seemed to be a message to me. I remember it well. It was a verse that says, *And be thou there until I bring thee word*—the words spoken by the Lord when he appeared in a dream to Joseph and told him to go down into Egypt with Mary and the Infant Jesus. It meant to me, *Stay where you are until you're told to move.* So I stayed on and [this was the second unexpected happening]

I met a nurse named Olive Rogers whom I eventually married. That, then, was *very* crucial in my life."

In 1940, after the evacuation of the British forces from Dunkirk, he volunteered for the army. They did not need more surgeons, and he was turned down. He then applied to the Colonial Office, specifying that he would like to work in West Africa and explaining that he wanted to go out there "with a Christian motive." Again he was turned down, this time for the reason, on paper, that he had lost an eye and therefore did not have enough sight for surgical work. The more likely explanation, he realized later, was that his motive alarmed the authorities. In those days the Colonial Service preferred men who were good company, who would fit in, who could hold their drink like gentlemen. Missionary types were suspect.

"Two days after the Colonial Office rejected me, I was reading the account in Exodus of the Israelites coming to the Red Sea; and their way was barred—they could not cross. And God said to Moses, *Speak unto the children of Israel, that they go forward,* in spite of the fact that they faced what seemed to be a total and impassable barrier. I felt that it was right for me: even though I had been turned down I was sure the way would open up again, just as it opened up for Moses. And I applied once more to the army, and I was accepted."

The next two years were spent in England. Then, on July 28, 1943, at a time when he was attached to an army hospital near Southampton, he took 48 hours' leave and married Olive. "We couldn't get a car, we couldn't get petrol, so we went away on our honeymoon by bus, straphanging all the way because the bus was full. When we arrived at the bus station in Midhurst, Sussex, we had to walk three miles to the hotel, carrying our suitcases, because there were no taxis."

Many honeymoon couples encounter troubles of this order, war or no war; they are part and parcel of traditional
honeymoon procedure, nerve-racking at the time but acquiring a patina as the years go by, so that they ultimately take
their place as gay and touching recollections of one's youth
and innocence. But the essential factor in this honeymoon
was that Denis Burkitt had found a wife who fully understood and fully shared his beliefs. In view of what developed
later this was of paramount importance, and he has expressed
it with great force: "I would not even have considered choos-
ing a life partner with whom I did not feel a unity at that
deeper level. In looking for a wife that was the first and absolute requirement, before anything else. I realize now how
exceedingly little we knew each other, yet how exceedingly
much I found in her which I did not know was there then.
Again, to me, it is an example of how, if in these matters
one seeks God's will, one gets abundant blessings out of it."

Then, almost at once, he was posted overseas. Denis and
Olive Burkitt were separated for the first two and a half years
of their married life.

He still wanted to go to West Africa. The army posted him to
East Africa. It was as if, wishing to go to New York, he were
taken instead to California, three thousand miles away. The
point is of some importance in a review of Denis Burkitt's
career: he did not choose East Africa; he was *sent* there, he
found himself there. He served first in Kenya, later in neighboring Somaliland; and his duty as surgical officer was to look
after African troops. For a while he was in Ceylon, then in
Singapore.

The most significant event in his overseas service occurred when, on a local leave, he went to stay with friends in
Uganda. Here, finally, he felt he had found his place. The

physical features of the country, its scenery, its climate, pleased him; furthermore, it was largely an *African* country rather than a *settler* country—the difference, before independence, was important. His friends seemed to be making a strong impact upon the people, in both a spiritual and a material sense; and he met Africans who impressed him very deeply with their dedication, their honesty, their positive Christian approach to life. He felt impelled to help, to lend a hand here, to do whatever he could for these people, and when he arrived home in 1946 the feeling was strongly rooted. His calling, specifically, was to return to Uganda and work there. Once again, in his own words, he experienced the certainty that this was God's will, this was what he was destined to do. It could not be ignored.

It could not be ignored, but there was another factor to be taken into account. During his absence Olive had continued working as a Sister in a hospital in Eastbourne. Now the war was over. Major Burkitt had returned from distant lands and had resumed his former identity as Mr. Denis Burkitt, a Fellow of the Royal College of Surgeons (Edinburgh); and Olive Burkitt, like any young wife, was longing to settle down, to have a home of her own, to raise a family. She had not the slightest desire to go to Uganda; it was the last place in the world she would have chosen. Her inclination was to settle down in England; and her husband was tempted to throw everything to the winds and settle down with her.

For both partners it was a difficult time. In the end he was unable to turn away from what was so strongly implanted in him: the absolute necessity to follow his calling. The question, ultimately, was not one of deciding rationally what was the best course of action in the given circumstances. It was the infinitely more formidable question of heeding God's will—whatever God's will happened to be and no matter what it involved. That, in all his actions, *must* be the deciding factor.

A new application was made to go out in the Colonial Service, and after five years as a surgeon in the army he could hardly be turned down on the grounds of inadequate sight. But he was asked rather pointedly by the head of the Colonial Office if he was prepared to do anything they requested of him; he answered yes, feeling that if he said he would only do surgery it would be a mockery of his belief that he had a vocation to work in Africa. The point, in his mind, was of considerable importance. "If you say you have a vocation—a calling, a summons to the service of God—and then lay down stipulations, it's rather hypocritical. So I told them, *I'm not much good at anything except surgery, but I'll try to do whatever you ask.*"

He was accepted. He was then informed that he would be leaving for Africa in six months; and he was also informed that his wife could not accompany him. In those days, so soon after the war, there was a shortage of housing, and Colonial Service officers simply had to wait until accommodation for their families became available. So, after being separated for two and a half years, Denis and Olive Burkitt, with their first child on the way, were faced with another separation for an unspecified length of time. "I had to say goodby to her again," Denis Burkitt recalls, "and it was one of the most difficult things I've ever had to do."

5

Bush Surgeon

The sea journey in 1946 took about a month. The route was becoming familiar to Burkitt: across the Bay of Biscay, through the Straits of Gibraltar into the Mediterranean, passing Malta and Crete on the way to Port Said, through the Red Sea and the Gulf of Aden, and down the Indian Ocean to Mombasa, the chief port of Kenya. Mombasa is hot, humid, steamy, and it still carries memories of the centuries of horror when it was a center of the Arab trade in ivory and slaves. It is prosperous today, with a population of 150,000; ten minutes in a cabin cruiser will take visitors to some of the most exciting deep-sea fishing in the world; its harbor is picturesque, its waterfront is picturesque, its people are picturesque; but it is tainted—it cannot shake off the past as Buchenwald will never shake off the past.

Postwar scarcities prevailed here, too. Burkitt, coming ashore after his month at sea, could not get a room for the night and slept in the lounge of a small hotel. Early in the morning—the first morning of his new life in Africa—he walked out of the hotel into the bush for a few minutes of solitude and prayer.

Then he went by train to Nairobi. One of his companions, not by choice, was a senior Colonial Service officer who was so drunk that the African stewards had to carry him to bed. Burkitt vividly remembers the man emptying his bladder on the carriage floor: "And I remember saying to myself, If this is the example England gives to Africa, may God help me to give something different." He had always abstained from drinking; this experience affected him deeply and strengthened his resolve to stay away from alcohol.

From Nairobi he went to Kampala, and then in a small pick-up truck to his station: Lira, the principal town of Lango District, which stretches north from an immense complex of lakes, rivers, and marshes. The district immediately to the west, Bunyoro, includes the Murchison Falls National Park and extends to Lake Albert and the Congo frontier; the district to the north, Acholi, reaches to the Sudan.

As the crow flies, Lira is about a hundred and fifty miles from Kampala, but the crow is presumed to go in a straight line across all the rivers and swamps, across Lake Kioga and Lake Kwania, whereas a small pick-up truck has to travel in an arc, skirting the lakes and crossing the Victoria Nile by ferry at Atura, thus adding about seventy miles to the distance. Burkitt had already spent more than a year in East Africa, and the town was scarcely any different from the mental picture he had formed of it before his arrival. The Indian population lived in its own quarter, the bazaar; the Africans for the most part lived outside the town itself; the Europeans lived in red-tiled or corrugated-iron houses around the golf course and the all-important club. No building was more than a single story high. The surrounding country was absolutely flat; the roads were of the usual red mud, bordered by tall elephant grass, and ran perfectly straight for miles on end. There was none of the lushness one associates with tropical Africa, no rain forest, no wild outbursting vegetation. Here the most common tree was the rather drab Borassus palm, which rattles in the breeze as if its leaves are made of tin, and has a swelling on its trunk as if it is permanently pregnant. Virtually all the large wild animals had been killed or driven away.

It was very backward when Burkitt first went there. "Out in the bush," he says, "most people still wore animal skins. They grew cotton, and lived on millet and sorghum and sweet potatoes; and they were very friendly." For a couple of days he was put up in a rest house. Then he was given his own house, and on the day he moved into it an African came to see him and said he would like to be Burkitt's houseboy. His name was Yusufu, and he remained with the Burkitt family for the next twenty years, until they left Uganda. His portrait, painted by one of the hospital sisters, hangs today in the dining room of the Burkitt's home in England.

Olive joined him, with their first child, Judy, six months later. Denis went to Mombasa to meet her. "She'd had a terrible journey coming out. The conditions were like a troopship. There were thirteen mothers and children in one cabin, all going down with various infectious fevers, and she thought she would never get our daughter off the boat alive. We came back most of the way by train, but the last part of the trip was in the pick-up truck; and she told me later that she was horrified to see that I had such a big staff just for myself. In those days, of course, it was a kindness to the people to take them on as staff. I had a cook, and a boy to help the cook, and a houseboy, and a boy to work in the garden; and when Olive came I engaged an ayah for her."

It was a pleasant life, despite the primitive conditions. "The toilet was just a bucket, emptied every day by an ox-wagon. We carried in the water for the bath in a four-gallon drum. The light was an Aladdin lamp, or a hurricane lamp. And we were very happy. It would never have done to have started in Kampala and then gone upcountry. It's far easier in life to begin with simple living and go on to something better, than to go the other way. . . . One didn't work excessive hours under those circumstances. We reported to the hospital at about eight o'clock in the morning. We took an hour for lunch, and finished work at about half past four. We were always on call, because there was nowhere to go." In addition to the medical officer there was the usual establishment, found on most upcountry stations: the agricultural officer, the forestry officer, the police officer, and the District Commissioner, each with his own little office and his own house. Altogether there were perhaps a dozen European families. Prisoners from the local jail kept the golf course spick and span, and the District Commissioner was looked upon as a sort of Great White Father of the area. Relations between the administration and the people were excellent. At no time was there any element of resentment, of hostility, of danger. The whites followed the traditional mode of colonial life: wives gathered for coffee in midmorning, returned home for lunch with husbands, regrouped for afternoon tea and tennis, went to the club afterward. It has been described in novels a thousand times, and each time you read about it you wonder how the people survived the process of going around and around in a circle.

For Burkitt (and this was undoubtedly true also for his

colleagues in their particular fields) boredom was the very least of his problems. At that time, England had a statistical ratio of one doctor for every thousand people. In Lira, assisted by a single African doctor, Burkitt looked after a population of considerably more than a quarter of a million. He was responsible for public health in the entire district. He was responsible for the schools. He was responsible for the hospital administration. And he was responsible, of course, for surgery. No cars were available when he first went out: he traveled everywhere by bicycle or, in special circumstances, by ambulance. Eventually he acquired his trusty Ford pick-up truck, which was ten years old and notable for having virtually no brakes. "But since the country is entirely flat," he says, quite reasonably, "and since every road is entirely straight, and since, also, there is no traffic, the pick-up truck was fairly safe because one always had a mile or so in which to glide to a stop."

The central hospital in Lira had a hundred beds, but scattered around Lango District there were about a dozen sub-dispensaries staffed by medical orderlies. Once a week Burkitt would go on safari, visiting them. "That was why I chose a pick-up truck. I would find among the patients at the sub-dispensaries some who definitely needed hospital treatment, and I would pile them in the back of the truck and bring them to the hospital. Then, when I went out again, I would fill up the back of the truck with patients who were ready to go home, and return with another truckload of patients who needed operations. At the same time I'd carry out drugs and any other supplies the dispensaries needed."

Occasionally he took Olive with him on safari overnight, and apart from almost being eaten to death by mosquitoes she survived these experiences very well. Later, she learned that the country around Lira was highly malarial. The climate was not too hot for Europeans: the temperature rarely went above 88°, never went below 72°. Given a refrigerator, which the Burkitts could not obtain in Lira because of postwar shortages, life would have been unshadowed. Even without a refrigerator they were happy and content.

In his first year at Lira, Burkitt increased the number of operations from seventeen to more than 600. By and large, the people were debilitated by chronic malaria, by hookworms, and by all the other infections and parasites that afflict the African in the bush. They were highly susceptible to tuberculosis and meningitis. Most of them were anemic. Hernias were common, due to three factors: incompetent surgery at birth, which leaves the child with a defective, protuberant navel; poor diet, both for children and adults, which results in a distended abdomen; and the picturesque habit of carrying heavy loads on the head, which puts great pressure on the spinal column, the pelvic muscles, and the abdominal wall. A great many of Burkitt's cases were hydroceles, a collection of fluid in the testicles often resulting in enormous distention. This, because he had to treat it so often, led to his first venture into geographic pathology—the study of the manner in which disease is affected by climate and geographical location; and he came up with a remarkable finding—in the eastern part of his district one man in three suffered from hydrocele, while in the western part the incidence dropped to 1 percent. This finding was never followed through, and why hydrocele should occur in such a peculiar pattern remains obscure. Fortunately (in a sense), hernias and hydrocele require what Burkitt terms "short" operations. Whenever possible he had to concentrate on procedures and treatment "where one is able to do the most good with the minimum expenditure of time, material and effort, because the circumstances are such that it is only possible to touch the fringe of all that needs to be done."

Injuries of various kinds helped to fill the hospitals and dispensaries. Mostly they were the outcome of fights—the free use of knives, pangas, bludgeons, and other simple weapons readily available in the bush. Severe bite wounds were frequent, and it is a remarkable fact that the hospital treated eight victims of human bites for every snakebite victim. Human bites can be exceedingly dangerous, even lethal, because of infection; on the other hand, there are few highly poisonous snakes in Uganda and snakebite deaths are relatively infrequent.

The Lira experience was to prove of immense value to Denis Burkitt. It strengthened his confidence in himself: when, a dozen times a day, you are confronted with decisions that mean life or death, you *must* have confidence in yourself, in your own values, your own judgment, otherwise you collapse inwardly, and probably outwardly, too. It gave him, also, an understanding of the problems faced by all upcountry doctors, in both government and mission hospitals. He had been in their shoes. He was one of them; and they could trust him.

The Colonial Office presumably had the right to send him anywhere they pleased. Fifteen months after he arrived in Lira they exercised their prerogative. In January 1948, he received a telegram informing him that he was posted to Mulago Hospital in the capital, Kampala.

The reasons for the transfer were perfectly valid (and even if they were not, Burkitt would still have had to comply with his orders). Mulago Hospital, which grew from the primitive hospitals started by Sir Albert Cook, was the center of the government hospital system in Uganda. Late in 1947 the senior surgeon had retired and returned to England, and as a consequence all surgery in the hospital was being done by the one surgeon who remained, Professor Ian McAdam. The pressure of work proved so great that he fell ill with an acute duodenal ulcer and a message was hastily sent to Burkitt requesting him to come down to Mulago and take over.

Mulago Hospital, named for the hill on which it stands, was then a collection of miscellaneous buildings, for the most part huts, which had grown up over the years in a fairly haphazard way. Hut was simply added to hut when a particular need arose. The war had curtailed any further growth, but by 1948 the hospital was enlarging its facilities once again. Separate units were formed for surgery, medicine, and gynecology, and in due course there was to be a further subdivision into what was probably the most important of all services for the African community, pediatrics.

In some ways Burkitt was not sorry to be transferred. Looking back on the time he spent in Lira, he felt duly grateful for being given the opportunity to turn his hand to so many different things. But his chief skill was as a surgeon, "and I had, perhaps, the selfish hankering to get back to surgery altogether. Not that I was particularly competent as a surgeon. . . . But I knew more about surgery than anything else."

The work load was far heavier than it had been at Lira. At the beginning there were only two qualified surgeons— McAdam and Burkitt, assisted by five or six junior doctors (today the surgical staff is more than sixty). The encouraging and exciting aspect of the situation when Burkitt arrived was that Mulago was growing in every sense, and it continued to grow: "I had the privilege and opportunity of growing with it. If you find yourself linked to a growing place, you are carried up with it as it grows. If you link up with a place that is going down, you tend to go down with it. From that point of view I was very fortunate." Within a couple of years a Department of Surgery was formed, and Sir John Croot was appointed Professor of Surgery. The medical side, with separate wards and facilities, was headed by a man whom Burkitt calls the best-known doctor in East Africa at that time, Dr. H. C. Trowell.

For ten years Burkitt worked at Mulago Hospital, heading one of the three surgical units—Professor Ian McAdam and Sir John Croot headed the other two—when, without any forewarning, the direction of his life was decisively changed. It was as if he were in a boat going up a broad river, and suddenly the boat turned away from the main stream and continued up a branch of the river he had never seen before. The actual event was nothing more than a common occurrence in the daily routine. Something of the same sort happened all the time.

One day—nobody can recall the precise date—Dr. Hugh Trowell asked Denis Burkitt if he would be kind enough to look at a patient in Ward One of the old Mulago Hospital.* There was nothing unusual about the request, there was no emergency. It was ordinary procedure—one doctor asking another doctor for an opinion. "I can't remember whether I

* A brief explanation may avoid confusion. The old Mulago Hospital is "the collection of huts" referred to earlier, although the main building was comparatively elaborate—a pavilion-type colonial structure, surmounted by a graceful little clock tower, looking rather like a primitive Howard Johnson's restaurant. The new Mulago Government Hospital, built to replace it, is one of the most impressive hospitals in the world, a striking example of modern hospital design.

was the surgeon on duty, or whether he just said to me in passing, *Denis, would you look at this patient for me.* Ward One was the children's ward, and we both had patients in it."

The patient Dr. Trowell asked Burkitt to look at was a boy aged about five. An ordinary small boy. What made him different from other small boys was that he had swellings in all four quadrants of his jaws—that is, swellings on both sides of the upper jaw, and swellings on both sides of the lower jaw.

The little boy's name was Africa. His parents gave him the name out of love and pride, perhaps, or because they could not think of any other name to give him. Other people in other lands might be called Walter Scott, or William Henry Ireland, or John Philip Holland; but this child's name was Africa, and he was undoubtedly very frightened at finding himself in Ward One of the old Mulago Hospital.

The best-known doctor in East Africa could not explain those four symmetrical jaw swellings; nor could the surgeon whose opinion had been requested. They could be sure of only one thing: little Africa would not live very long.

"Ever since I came to Mulago in 1948 we—the other medical officers and myself—had seen tumors of the jaws in children," Denis Burkitt now says. "They were cancers. We cut them out.

"But this boy had swellings on both sides of both jaws, which was unusual. I didn't think it was a tumor—it made no *sense* as a tumor, because nobody is likely to have four tumors at once. It didn't make sense as an infection, either.

"I examined him very carefully, made some notes, and took some photographs—I always carried two cameras, one for black and white and one for color photographs. Afterwards I discussed the case with Hugh Trowell, and I told him I didn't know what it was. We had tissue sent out for section (that is, for examination under the microscope) but this didn't help us very much; and we just felt—Hugh and I—that we didn't know the diagnosis. This isn't as peculiar as it sounds. It happens often. One is frequently meeting things one can't pin down.

"In a country like England you can turn to all sorts of experts for their opinion and advice, but in Uganda in those days there weren't many experts to whom we could turn. There were conditions which you recognized because you saw them fairly frequently: you knew, *This is this* by what it looked like, or what it felt like, but you had no name for it. You couldn't say exactly *what* it was until somebody found an organism, or detected something or other, that caused it.

"And the jaw condition on this little boy, Africa, was just one of the queer, unidentified things we came across. It was interesting. But neither Hugh Trowell nor I could say with certainty what it was."

Then, only a few weeks later, when he was visiting the district hospital in Jinja, on the northern shore of Victoria Nyanza, fifty miles from Kampala, he happened to glance out of the window of one of the wards; and there, on the grass, was another child with a fat, swollen face. Burkitt hurried outside and found that he was not mistaken. "It was just the same as the mouth of the little boy I had seen in Mulago Hospital. I took photographs again, and I made notes. And I began thinking about these things seriously."

So, early in 1957, the drama began.

6

Interlude:
A Different Pyramid

Hugh Carey Trowell takes a place at the very outset of the Burkitt story by virtue of a few concerned words spoken to a colleague. The results were to be startling. But Dr. Trowell also has a place of his own in the history of medicine in East Africa, and his contributions to the well-being of millions of human beings are of tremendous importance.

London, not Dublin, was Hugh Trowell's background. He trained at St. Mary's Hospital from 1923 to 1928, did house jobs for a year, and experienced the spiritual call to go out to Africa. The wise men he consulted urged him to be sensible. He was told: *You have a great future here.* And he was solemnly warned: *The hospitals are very bad out there. You will be unable to do any decent work, and you will go with loose women, and you will take to drinking whisky, and after twenty years you will come home a total wreck.*

He married the day after he finished his house jobs. His

C

wife, Margaret, was a student at the Slade School of Art in Bloomsbury: she shared his beliefs, religious and humanitarian. Soon after they were married Hugh went out to Kenya in the Colonial Medical Service and was posted to a new hospital upcountry, about sixty miles from Nairobi—so new and primitive that there was not even a road leading to it. His wife accompanied him, and in this wilderness their first child was born.

Patients were few, for the simple reason that the Africans were utterly terrified of the white newcomers who—it was well known—ate the livers and other organs of anyone foolish enough to go to them for treatment. In addition to a lack of patients there was a lack of drugs, a lack of equipment, a lack of facilities, and Dr. Trowell (who can now look back and comment gently, "I was probably a difficult youngster") criticized the authorities so sharply that he expected to be sent home. The authorities, however, seemed impressed by the young man's spirit. After six months he was recalled to Nairobi and put in charge of a new project for training African medical orderlies, which raised quite unexpected problems—"the orderlies all thought they were going to be doctors the day after they started their training, and they went on strike because we wouldn't issue them stethoscopes."

He remained in Nairobi for nearly six years, and during this time he became aware of an unusual disease of children —not the disease that aroused Denis Burkitt's interest several years later but something else. He has written a searing account of it: "No one wanted the old K.A.R. [King's African Rifles] Hospital in Nairobi, so I was given it. In sullen mood I went into the corrugated iron building; it was dark, it was full of bed lice, the children were all crying, but many of them had brown hair although they were African babies and many of them had swollen legs with edema. On walking through the ward at night, lit by one hurricane lantern, one would hear the low moan of the children dying; we did not know why they were dying, but it was Kwashiorkor. So there, as far as I am concerned, it all started. The 400-bedded hospital had one water tap; during all my six years it never had a microscope; no African could speak English; we could not even examine urine, stool, or blood slide in the hospital, everything went to a laboratory situated over a mile away. We only knew that when the baby developed black spots on the skin it was going to die. Then one day I surprised my wife by saying that I felt fairly certain I was dealing with a new disease. Its outstanding sign was the brown hair, the swollen legs of edema, but this is where the trouble started. There are so many causes for edema, all sorts of heart diseases, kidney diseases and blood diseases caused edema. Might not some recognized disease be there and missed? You could miss a lot, believe me, in the old Ward Five of the Nairobi K.A.R. Hospital."

It was indeed a new disease, and a particularly fearsome one. Unknown to Trowell then, an English missionary doctor in West Africa, Cicely Williams, had observed the same conditions in the children in her hospital, and it was she who one day learned from one of her nurses that the disease was called kwashiorkor. Cicely Williams asked, "What does 'kwashiorkor' mean?" The nurse explained, "It means the sickness that the older child gets when the next baby is born." And, according to Dr. Ann Dally in her biography, *Cicely: The Story of A Doctor*, Cicely Williams exclaimed, "My God, I believe that's the explanation." She had remembered the psalm: *I refrain my soul, and keep it low, like a child that is weaned from his mother: yea, my soul is even as a weaned child.*

The work of Cicely Williams and Hugh Trowell and,

later, other doctors, was to lead to the understanding of what the World Health Organization called "the most widespread and severe nutritional disorder known to medical science." It has become only too familiar in recent years as a result of the ghastly war fought between the Nigerians and the Biafrans. Those children with the fleshless skulls and bloated abdomens are in the terminal stage of kwashiorkor, and it is no longer the weaning disease but the disease of relentless and disgraceful fratricide.

In reasonably peaceful tropical areas it is due to protein deficiency, often the result of a child being weaned because the mother is again pregnant, and being put on a diet which contains insufficient protein to meet the demands of early growth. In tropical areas ravaged by war, it is still due to a lack of protein, as a result of deliberate starvation, of unforgiveable human viciousness.

In 1935 Hugh Trowell and his family left Kenya for Uganda, and he took up new duties at Mulago Hospital. "It had some ten wards built of corrugated iron," he says. "The floors were mud, the roofs were grass. By the time I arrived these had more or less been replaced by huts with concrete floors. There were facilities for doing post mortems, a small laboratory where blood slides for malaria could be prepared; but you couldn't do any advanced biochemistry such as tests for blood proteins or blood sugar."

In Kenya there had been a rigid belief that no African could become a doctor; at best, he could only reach the level of a male nurse. Uganda was rather more enlightened, a legacy of the teaching of Sir Albert Cook and other medical missionaries. The mission hospitals, consequently, had gone ahead and were training what was vaguely termed "a doctor kind of person," more advanced than male nurses or medical orderlies but still far from a qualified physician.

"It was a very pleasant tropical setting," Dr. Trowell recalls. "African nationalism had not yet come to the fore. We weren't overwhelmed by large and complex instruments. Most of us had some disease we were chasing—mine was kwashiorkor. The white community remained apart, but some of us felt this shouldn't continue indefinitely, and we started to entertain some of the Africans in our home—it was slightly nerve-racking because if we were caught we would have been in serious trouble. The Africans couldn't speak English, and even if you were able to engage them in conversation you would have had to talk about goats, and crops, and the things that interested them.

"Early on it was difficult to get the Africans into the hospitals. We would go out into the markets, and we would take medicines with us and give them to the people; we'd leave the car in the market and if somebody was very ill we'd tell them to go and sit in the car so that we could examine them a little more carefully. They were very suspicious. They thought we were poisoning them. They had their own system of medicine—witch doctors who were not only medicine men but holy men of a sort, having great power: power over life and death."

During this time Margaret Trowell was marking out her own path. She had become very interested in the African's potential for art, and more or less as a hobby she had begun to give art lessons on the back veranda of her home. In due course this grew into a full-fledged art school. Her husband says of her: "In a strange way she released their artistic powers. She said to the Africans, *No, don't copy us, just have fun with paint and paper and get on with your own things.* She was also in charge of the museum; she collected African masks, and carvings, and weapons, and wrote about them, making us realize that they were really great works of art in their own right and that they should be a source of pride and inspiration to the African people." Today, Margaret Trowell is recognized as one of the outstanding authorities on African art and her books are known all over the world. As a tribute to her work, the art school in Makerere College was given her name when she retired—the Margaret Trowell School of Fine Art.

The discovery of kwashiorkor was not instantly acclaimed as a triumph of medicine. In West Africa, Cicely Williams became seriously ill as a result of her intensive study of the problem, and eventually accepted an appointment in Southeast Asia (where she was imprisoned by the Japanese during the war in the Pacific and suffered bitter hardships, including prolonged starvation, a subject on which she was a world authority). Hugh Trowell, in East Africa, was unable to define the problem in his own mind, and, hampered by inadequate scientific facilities, was assailed by people "who thought I was taking the thing too far."

Then, during World War II, Professor Harold Himsworth, at the time Professor of Medicine at University College, London, was asked by the British government to describe what diseases would occur in the British Isles if Britain lost the war. There was nothing academic about this exercise. Nazi submarines were taking an enormous toll of British shipping, destroying vast amounts of the imported foodstuffs that were essential to Britain's survival; and Nazi strategy, clearly, was to starve the British people into submission.

Since Britain could not import enough meat and would be unable to catch enough fish, and since most of her cattle would be killed so that pastures could be ploughed up for wheat, Himsworth could be certain that there would be a shortage of protein.

The first step, obviously, was to investigate the effects of protein shortage.

He induced protein malnutrition in rats and found that in addition to the expected symptoms—loss of weight, physical weakness, and so on—the liver of these animals was invaded and seriously damaged by excessive amounts of fat. Hugh Trowell, learning of Himsworth's work, sent him specimens of liver tissue taken from children who had died of kwashiorkor, showing similar evidence of excessive fatty deposits; and, in Trowell's words, Himsworth became very excited. His experimental disease, induced in rats in England, was actually occurring in human beings in East Africa, and he had a decisive answer to his question, at least as far as it affected young children. If Britain lost the war, the resultant shortage of protein would cause severe malnutrition and this could be expected to bring about a widespread condition similar to tropical kwashiorkor.

The mechanism of the disease was still unknown and there was no theory to account for its strange effects. Giving protein-rich foods to a child suffering from severe kwashiorkor would not necessarily change the course of his illness. You could virtually pour good food into him and he would still die. Why was protein starvation largely irreversible? Why couldn't a starved child be restored to health if he was given ample amounts of the proteins and vitamins he had been denied?

The answer was found by chance (or by the good fortune that seems to attend certain people) soon after World War II came to an end. Britain then had large stocks of powdered milk left over, and Trowell, through the Colonial Office, ordered supplies to be sent to him in Kampala to feed his kwashiorkor patients.

When the supplies arrived, Trowell's assistant came to him in great agitation and informed him that instead of powdered *whole* milk he had been sent *skimmed* milk.

At this, Hugh Trowell—normally the mildest and gentlest of men—flew into a tremendous rage. He was convinced that the bureaucrats in London were attempting to foist on him something they wanted to get rid of: processed milk, which had little nutritional value. But it appeared that the substitution might well have been arranged by higher authorities, for the children dying of kwashiorkor actually *thrived* on skimmed milk, and many of the symptoms of their disease were reversed. It was marvelous; and it seemed to make no sense. The children rejected whole milk, with its high nutritional value, but they willingly accepted skimmed milk.

Now, skimmed milk is milk from which the cream has been removed. Cream is largely butterfat. The digestion of fats, proteins, and starches is dependent upon the special secretion manufactured by the pancreas, which is called the pancreatic juice. This was the clue to the problem: kwashiorkor, among other things, causes the pancreas to become defective, so that there is a reduction in the activity of the pancreatic juice. Because of this failure the sick children were unable to digest whole milk with its high fat content, and the fat was deposited in the liver. Fat-free skimmed milk, on the other hand, provided the children with the nourishment they needed so desperately and gave them hope of a speedy recovery.

So kwashiorkor, which throughout the history of mankind must have affected the destinies of untold millions of human beings, ceased to be a mystery, although it still remains a severe problem. But, unquestionably, the work of

Cicely Williams and Hugh Trowell will in due course benefit
the inhabitants of every tropical nation in the world. They
were the true pioneers, the first not just to *see* the problem
but to *observe* it. The solution seemed to come by accident,
yet on this score it is worth recalling C. G. Jung's dictum:
There are no accidents.

In 1947 the British government was disturbed by reports
of serious unrest among porters working on the railways in
East Africa, and a board of inquiry was set up to look into
the situation. Dr. Trowell was appointed to review the medical aspects. He found that the porters' living conditions were
wretched, and he reported in the strongest terms that
changes were essential, the men must be fed better, must be
given better housing, must be given some hope for the
future. "I was appalled," he says, "by their aggressive, rebellious spirit; and this was in fact the beginning of the trouble
that erupted as the Mau Mau movement a year or so later."

There was a bonus. While he was traveling to Nairobi on
this mission he first met Denis Burkitt. "We were in the same
carriage on the train. We merely talked for a few hours, but
Denis made quite an impression on me. I thought, This is a
very keen man. We didn't discuss it much but I recognized
him to be a sincere Christian and I recognized, too, that he
would have what I call a warm attitude to the Africans. Not
everybody out there had it. He certainly would be one of
those who would be humane and fair."

So a friendship began. As far as medical history is concerned its most significant moment occurred ten years later
when Denis Burkitt entered Ward One of the old Mulago
Hospital at Dr. Trowell's request to examine a little boy
named Africa.

Like other physicians, Trowell had occasionally seen this

C*

condition in the past. Once, in 1935, when he was on safari to the islands of Lake Victoria, inspecting the population for evidence of sleeping sickness, he came across a little boy with "lumps" on the jaws. "I can't remember much about it except that I thought it was a peculiar complaint, and I told the boy, *I can't treat you here, you must come back to Mulago with me.* I didn't know what the disease was, because it wasn't one lump, which might be called an ordinary cancer, but several lumps. Vaguely, at the back of my mind, was the knowledge that the children out here had these lumps: one encountered them from time to time, one would ask surgeons to see them but nobody could throw much light on the trouble. When another case turned up in 1957 I asked Denis to look at it. I don't think I asked him in any deliberate way —it was just his turn to see surgical cases that week. Later, I remember him saying, *If you see any more of these cases, do let me know;* and I think we saw two or three of them in the next few months."

When Burkitt was posted to Mulago Hospital in 1948 he was still, in the professional sense, a young man. In order of seniority he was the third, or junior, member of the surgical team, and he was not expected to do the more elaborate and difficult surgical operations. His experience was of a different order from that of Professor Croot or Professor McAdam, both of whom came to Mulago after long connections with English teaching schools: John Croot had served for many years in the Department of Surgery at Bristol, Ian McAdam —a very forceful personality—had made a great name for himself at Edinburgh.

"Denis Burkitt," Trowell says, "was rather quiet and un-assuming, not at all the conventional picture of an incisive and purposeful surgeon. But when my son needed an opera-tion—it wasn't anything major—I was glad Denis performed it. If you had asked him, soon after he came to Mulago, *Are you ever going to be the Professor of Surgery here?* he would have said, *Oh, no, no. I'm very happy to be at Mulago Hospital, working with Africans, helping to train them, and so on. But Ian McAdam and the others are ahead of me.*

"The point is that he had, and still has, a great capacity to *pursue.* It's a temperamental gift which also links on to his religious beliefs. He was never obtrusive about his religion, he would never buttonhole people or indulge in great and elaborate theological discussions, and he had a great respect for anybody whose views differed from his: he was very charitable in his dealings with others."

Hugh and Margaret Trowell left Kampala in 1958 to return home. His work on kwashiorkor had resulted in extraordinary difficulties and in quite unexpected repercussions. For example, Communist agents attempted to contact him, hoping they could persuade him to say that kwashiorkor in Africa was due to colonialism, despite the established fact that the disease had been occurring for untold centuries throughout the tropics and elsewhere. (It was common in the Middle Ages, before the agricultural revolution in Europe; and there is a statue in a Florentine church which shows the Infant Christ with the big potbelly and swollen legs that are typical of the disease.) Trowell says, "We started by looking at the apex of an enormous pyramid. We didn't know how far down the base of the pyramid was, but in the end we began to realize that the majority of children in some parts of Africa and tropical Asia and tropical America have (at least) a mild degree of this disease. For a time we couldn't get agreement with the pathologists that this was a disease in its own right, so we couldn't find out why our children were dying; we couldn't get agreement with the biochemists, so we couldn't cure the thing. Now, looking back, I think that any idea—if it's really big—must be baptized with cold water. If the infant survives its baptism, it will thrive. . . .

"We have to ask why, in the world's history, the wheat eaters, or the cereal eaters, or those who had milk and meat, were able to create civilizations, whereas the people who had yams and cassava and all the other protein-deficient foods were unable to produce a civilization. I began to see that civilizations seldom arose in the tropics because the people failed to solve two problems: how to store calories, and how to get protein-rich food to growing children. Today this is possible, not by labeling any tropical food as bad, for they are all good and reflect the beneficence of Creation, but by adding other foods which can be stored, and are easily cooked, and are rich in protein.

"For me, it all started with babies crying in the night."

After his arrival in England he retired from medicine; he took holy orders, and he is now the Rev. Dr. Hugh Carey Trowell, vicar of Stratford-sub-Castle, in Salisbury. He has earned his place in history; and he can look at Denis Burkitt with understanding and with affection. "I know Denis terribly well," he says. "But if anybody had told me, *This is a man who is going to make a discovery of international importance,* I should have said no. He was too quiet, too modest. And I would have been wrong. The gifts which really land a major thing are humility, and perseverance, and seeing things fresh, and perhaps not taking a too exalted view of your own capacities. And, nearly always, the great discoveries start with just a tin can and a piece of string."

7

Invitation to a Safari

The doctors in Mulago Hospital could not save little Africa. In Jinja Hospital they could not save the other little boy who was suffering from the same disease. And so their parents came for them, in deep distress, bringing them great masses of fresh flowers, and carried them away to be laid to rest in the proper place and in the proper manner. It is a sight you see every day in any African hospital: the grieving parents in their best clothes, the motionless little body, the masses of flowers. Too many children die in Africa, of too many diseases.

The outcome was always the same, it was absolutely inevitable: all children with this peculiar disease, marked by heavily swollen jaws, died within six to twelve weeks after the illness became apparent. No drug—except to some slight extent the deadly war gas, nitrogen mustard—slowed the course of the disease. Surgery—and by its nature it was harsh and disfiguring surgery—gave only a brief respite. Young children between the ages of, say, two and ten grow at an astonishing rate. If by some terrible mischance they develop a malignancy it will grow as fast as the child's general rate of growth, and often a great deal faster. These jaw tumors grew very rapidly indeed. They doubled themselves in about forty-eight hours, and a young child could not live with them for more than about three months.

But why had a disease with such unmistakable symptoms failed to attract attention until 1957? Was it a new disease which was only now afflicting human beings; or was it a disease that had suddenly begun to occur with greater frequency; or had it, up to this time, been overlooked?

Anybody who has lived in Africa, even briefly, will have been touched by the tenderness that African parents show their children. The ancient social system works very well in this respect: families stay together, children are prized and receive infinite love from father and mother and all the other members of the particular group in which they live.

In these circumstances, the jaw tumors are not likely to be ignored. They first manifest themselves by loosened teeth, swollen and painful gums. Then, because of their rapid growth, the tumors become larger and more evident, and the child begins to suffer serious discomfort. The alarmed parents would then set out to seek help, if necessary walking twenty, thirty, or even fifty miles to the nearest hospital. Buses now run between the larger towns in East Africa and bicycles are abundant; but often, in the more remote areas, people have no money for a long bus ride and they walk from one place to another, plodding along the side of the red mud roads in single file. A woman taking her sick child to a hospital many miles away may carry him in her arms, at the same time carrying another child on her back or feeding at her breast, and balancing a bundle of her possessions on her head.

Over the years, then, most children with jaw tumors reached a hospital. They were seen by doctors or by nurses or by medical orderlies. They received treatment. They died. And this has been going on for a very long time. Sir Albert Cook had described the condition in his notebooks, calling it a sarcoma—a term used for a certain type of tumor. "Sarcomas are common in Africa," he wrote in 1902, "particularly sarcomas of the jaw." Hugh Trowell had seen them, first on Lake Victoria, later at Mulago; and other doctors in East Africa had seen them and drawn attention to them without arousing any great interest.

As for Denis Burkitt, during his fifteen months at Lira he must certainly have encountered a case or two, and quite certainly he encountered several cases during the years he was at Mulago. Somehow or other these cases did not arouse him, they did not produce any great inner excitement. He himself says, "I *must* have been seeing the tumor in those first ten years in Africa, but we weren't recognizing it. There's a great difference between seeing a thing and observing a thing, and unless you actually look for it, it can pass you unnoticed."

What occurred to Denis Burkitt, then, was no sudden vision, no sudden flash of inspiration, nothing as dramatic and immediate as Sir Isaac Newton's apple falling in the orchard. After ten years, so he says, he woke up to something that had been there all along. One has to remember, though, that Burkitt maintained a heavy schedule of surgery, that he had to concern himself with the endless details which are an inescapable part of hospital routine, and that he took his responsibility toward his patients very seriously: he cared about them, he worried about them.

Yet it is clear that the child in Ward One of Mulago Hospital and the child playing on the grass outside Jinja Hospital rarely left his thoughts. He could have left the problem where it was, of course, merely noting that he had run across something unusual—symmetrical swellings on both sides of the upper and lower jaws; but his interest was stirred, he was compelled to go on.

The first step was to examine the records of all children who had been treated at Mulago for jaw tumors.

Next, he went over the records of all children who had been treated for tumors of any kind.

And, as new patients with the disease came to the hospital, he looked at them more closely.

As a rule, a malignant growth originates in one particular place in the body. In other words, it will at first involve only a single site, it will have a single focus. For example, it may first appear in a kidney, as an almost imperceptible colony of malignant cells, and there it will continue to grow to an appreciable size. This—the original growth—is known as the primary tumor; and a primary tumor alone can often be treated successfully by surgery or radiotherapy.

As the tumor grows, unfortunately, some malignant cells may migrate to other parts of the body, to a lung, perhaps, or to the liver; and they may initiate new growths, which are known as secondary tumors. When a malignancy spreads in this fashion it becomes exceedingly serious because treatment is far more difficult.

Burkitt uncovered a strange state of affairs in these children with the jaw tumors. "When I examined them more carefully I found that whenever we had a jaw tumor *there would be another tumor elsewhere*. The jaw tumor was not an isolated occurrence. There might also be tumors of the long bones, or of the thyroid, the kidneys, the ovaries, and so on."

The significance of this finding was that *the same disease* could appear in many different forms. It might manifest itself as a jaw tumor. But it might manifest itself without involving the jaws at all. It might first become apparent as an abdominal tumor, or as an ovarian tumor, or as a kidney tumor; nevertheless, these were all manifestations of the same disease, coming to the surface at different places in different children. And when more than one tumor was found in a child, they were all part of what might be called a multiple or multifocal tumor.

In the past each of these tumors had been classified as a separate entity. Now, with the recognition that they were all the same tumor—no matter where they first showed up—an accurate identification became possible. For a time it was thought that they might be neuroblastomas, but two of Burkitt's colleagues, Professor J. N. P. Davies and Dr. G. T. O'Conor, showed that the strange multiple tumor was a form of lymphoma. *

* The terms "neuroblastoma" and "lymphoma" need, and deserve, a rather more detailed explanation.

A *neuroblastoma* is a tumor arising from early forms of nerve cells. It frequently originates in one of the adrenal glands (which sit like a cap over each kidney) and may spread from there to the cranium, the liver, lungs, lymph nodes, and bones.

A *lymphoma* is a malignancy affecting the lymphatic system, which consists of lymphatic vessels, lymph nodes, and lymphoid (or lymphatic) tissue.

The *lymphatic system* is a circulatory system similar in many ways to the circulating blood system. It carries the lymph,

"In those days," Burkitt says, "we used to have a staff meeting on Saturday mornings, when the physicians and surgeons and gynecologists met together and one of them would present for discussion any special work he was doing. It was at one of these Saturday morning meetings in Mulago Hospital that I first presented this information about a tumor of

---

which bathes all the tissues of the body. Lymph is a transparent liquid, resembling blood plasma, containing varying numbers of white blood cells and a few red blood cells.

The *lymphatic* vessels branch throughout the body like the blood vessels. They are somewhat fragile, with thinner walls than the veins.

Lymph nodes are small bean-like structures composed of a mesh, or network, of tissue containing fixed white blood cells (as distinct from the free-moving white blood cells in the circulating blood). The network within a lymph node acts as a filter, trapping any solid particles that may have entered the lymph, and engulfing harmful organisms such as bacteria. In many infections, the lymph nodes become swollen and painful, and can be felt as "glands" under the angle of the jaw, under the armpits, or in the groin, but they are also found in the inner side of the knees and the elbows, and in great profusion in the linings of the digestive tract, the liver, the respiratory passages, and the cavity containing the heart.

Lymphoid tissue is composed of a network similar to the lymph nodes and acts in much the same way. The tonsils and the adenoids are composed of lymphoid tissue; so is much of the spleen, the thymus and the appendix.

Lymph nodes and lymphoid tissue form a vital part of the body's defense against infection. They compose the *reticuloendothelial system*, which simply means the system of networks lining the interior surface of the blood vessels, lymph vessels, and cavities in the bone marrow, the spleen, the liver, and other organs.

the jaw with deposits in other parts of the body. Everyone was very interested."

At the end of 1957, Dr. George Oettlé visited Kampala, and by good fortune Denis Burkitt met him and thus had an opportunity to talk to him.

George Oettlé was an outstandingly brilliant young man. At the time of this meeting he was (at the age of thirty-six) Director of the Cancer Research Unit of the National Cancer Association of South Africa, at the South African Institute for Medical Research, and he had done remarkable work on various malignancies that seem to occur with uncommon frequency in some regions of Africa—cancer of the liver, for example, and cancer of the esophagus.*

He was obviously just the man to be consulted about the strange tumor that had caught Burkitt's attention. "I met him

---

* What is of particular interest is that, like Denis Burkitt and other people in this story, he was deeply religious. A few words by a colleague, Professor J. F. Murray, deserve to be quoted: "Critical to a degree, he used his brilliant mind to test and evaluate every statement he encountered and every set of facts uncovered in the course of his research. Nothing irritated him more than loose or slovenly thinking, and he delighted in the application of logic to the assessment of his research findings. . . . He had a profound knowledge of the Bible and was a man of deep and unshakeable faith in the Providence of God. Despite his brilliant mind, his great scientific achievements, and his research ability he was a humble and lovable man. . . . No one could be long in the presence of George Oettlé without realizing that this was a man whose every thought and action was coloured and determined by Christian love and faith."

George Oettlé died in November 1968, after emergency heart surgery. His contribution to medical science was immense. A further reference to him will be found on p. 233, in Mr. Burkitt's diary.

at the hospital," Burkitt says. "I showed him my photographs and slides. I said, *I am interested in this problem,* and I told him what I was doing about it and asked for his ideas. He was interested in the histology (that is, the microscopic structure of the tissues of the tumor) and he was interested in the cases."

Oettlé was interested for a good reason. When he finished looking at the photographs and slides he told Burkitt, simply but with authority, that this tumor did not occur in South Africa.

Most people would have accepted it as a straightforward statement of fact: *This tumor does not occur in South Africa.* But once again Burkitt reacted in his own characteristic way; he mulled over Oettlé's comment and began to ask himself some new questions.

The distance from Kampala to Johannesburg, as the crow flies, is about 1,800 miles, and the crow would have to fly over a number of different countries—from Uganda over Tanzania, Zambia, Mozambique, Rhodesia, and Botswana, skirting the Congo and Malawi. It would also fly over the great expanse of Lake Victoria, Lake Tanganyika, and (if it lost its bearings slightly) Lake Nyasa. It would miss the snowcapped, cloud-covered Mountains of the Moon, but it would have to cross the Muchinga Mountains, and it would see numerous great rivers—the Ruaha, the Luangwa, the Zambesi, the Limpopo, and many others. There would be all kinds of terrain—marshes, hills, forests, veldt.

Now, Burkitt said to himself, if the tumor occurs commonly (or relatively commonly) here in Uganda, and it does not occur at all some two thousand miles away in South Africa, *where does it stop?*

Clearly it had to stop somewhere between Uganda and South Africa. There had to be a line (he called it *an edge*) dividing tumor territory from non-tumor territory. *Here,* children could have the disease; *there,* children did not have the disease. If such an edge could be found it would be of great interest, of superlative interest, because it might provide some clues to this tumor—environmental clues, hereditary clues, dietary clues, anything.

And, as it happened, *Where does it stop?* turned out to be one of the most stimulating questions in medical history.

Burkitt then took an immense step forward, and boldly applied for a grant to support his research. Cancer research is a costly business, and tens or hundreds of thousands of dollars may be required to start a project and keep it going. Burkitt obtained his grant: the impressive sum of £15 (about forty dollars). He used it for printing and mailing 1,200 leaflets illustrated with his own photographs of children with the tumor. "We obtained addresses from everybody we could. Then we sent the leaflets to government and mission doctors throughout Africa, with a little questionnaire asking, *How long have you worked in your hospital, and have you seen this condition?"*

This preliminary work, as he calls it, went on for about three years. "It was a part-time hobby, because I was employed full time as a government surgeon. But, at a guess, I might have had three to four hundred replies from different parts of Africa. Whenever I spoke at a conference I would get addresses from people. I would meet Dr. Brown, who knew Dr. Smith, who worked at such and such a place, and I would write to him. It wasn't all done at once, and the answers came in dribs and drabs."

At the end of the three years something valuable had been accomplished. On the wall of his office hung several maps. The information provided by the doctors who answered his questionnaire was plotted on these maps by means of colored pins. "We couldn't afford fourpence each [4¢] for mapping pins," Burkitt says, "so I painted the heads of drawing pins myself in different colors to distinguish the different tumors."

The colored drawing pins showed that there was a belt right across equatorial Africa where this children's tumor was common. There was also a sort of tail hanging down East Africa from Kenya to Mozambique.

So the tumor had a pattern of its own. It was obeying certain laws. It was not a haphazard occurrence.

A map may provide an immense amount of information, but it is only a special kind of document. A painted drawing pin is only a kind of symbol, and it cannot talk to you in detail about what it represents. The obvious thing for Denis Burkitt to do next was to go out and look at the situation himself, and he began to plan a trip which—he hoped—would clarify the mystery. "I said to myself, we have to find an edge. If we can find an edge to the belt, that might be the place to look for some environmental factor related to the tumor."

There was little point looking for an edge north of the belt: here one entered the bleak, unpopulated areas of the Sudan and Ethiopia. Due east and due west, the tumor belt went all the way to the sea. In the Congo medical services had been hopelessly disrupted, and any European might find himself in trouble. The best hope was the tail hanging down from the eastern end of the belt, a thickly populated area with many hospitals.

At the outset he fancied that he would buy a secondhand Volkswagen and drive down to South Africa alone, visiting hospitals on the way. After he had given this some thought he realized that it would be much too tiring, and that companionship was essential on such a long trip.

One of his best friends, Dr. E. H. (Ted) Williams, director of a mission hospital near Arua, in northeast Uganda, happened to be visiting Kampala, and Burkitt asked him if he would be prepared to join the safari.

Dr. Williams was not at all happy about it. He was due to go on leave to England; there were various family complications; and he replied, "I don't know if I can, Denis." Burkitt said, "I wish you would," and Dr. Williams returned to Arua, thought about it, then wrote to Burkitt saying he would go. Mrs. Williams would travel to England by herself and stay there while her husband went on safari to South Africa.

"But I felt," Burkitt says, "that there ought to be three people, because if you invite only one, and he drops out through sickness or for some other reason, you are left alone and the whole thing collapses. If there are two others, and one has to return home, you can still continue."

The third man to be invited was Cliff Nelson, a Canadian. He had been in government medical service in Uganda, and when his contract expired he joined Dr. Williams' mission (the Africa Inland Mission, which is predominantly American, with headquarters in Brooklyn).

So, with a full complement, Burkitt settled down to planning the safari in detail.

8

The Long Safari

The immediate plans called for a safari of no less than ten thousand miles. The immediate problem was how to pay for it. Again, good fortune came to Denis Burkitt's aid. One day Sir Harold Himsworth (who had been knighted since the war, when he and Hugh Trowell communicated in high excitement about protein deficiency, and was now Director of the Medical Research Council in London) walked into Burkitt's office and asked him about his current work. Burkitt described the projected trip to South Africa. Sir Harold asked, "How much money do you need?" Burkitt was taken aback: "Very tentatively—I was afraid to ask for too much—I said I was terribly anxious, if it was at all possible, to get together about £100 [$280] for this safari. And Sir Harold said, *I think I'll make it £150*. But then, when he went back to England he sent me £250."

This was Burkitt's third research grant. He had originally received £15 from government funds and then another £10, all of which had long since been spent on leaflets and

74

postage stamps, not to mention drawing pins. With £250 from Sir Harold Himsworth, Burkitt must have felt he had come into a fortune, and he forthwith commissioned Dr. Williams to try to find a suitable secondhand car.

Now, Dr. Ted Williams has an affinity—among other affinities—for mechanical things: for shortwave radios, and cameras, and plumbing fixtures, and—particularly important at this juncture—cars. He understands these dumb objects, and it is very possible that they are aware that he understands them, for they tend to respond to him. And one of the reasons Denis Burkitt was eager to have his company on the safari (among other reasons) was Ted Williams' magic way with automobiles. "He could change a big end bearing," Burkitt says with pride, "while you were having a cup of coffee. He could do anything to a motor car in any circumstances; and that, of course, is invaluable." To which Dr. Williams retorts, "Not true. Just typical Burkitt blarney."

The Simba were on the rampage in the Congo; mission hospitals were being burned down, missionaries were being slaughtered. One member of the Africa Inland Mission in the Congo was fortunate enough to get away unharmed and managed to reach Ted Williams' hospital just across the border in northern Uganda. He was driving a 1953 Ford Jubilee stationwagon—an American model, with left-hand drive—which had already covered some 45,000 miles of the indescribably appalling Congo roads. Dr. Williams was able to acquire it for £250.

The Jubilee was then given a thorough overhaul and two spare tires were attached to the roof. Since car thieves are just as active in Darkest Africa as elsewhere—perhaps even more so—Dr. Williams followed his usual practice of installing a secret ignition switch. Later, somewhere in the middle of Tanzania, after a day's drive during which they passed a total of two cars, one of which was wrapped around a tree, the Jubilee suddenly stopped dead. Dr. Williams' secret ignition switch had let him down; and apart from a flat tire at nine thousand miles and a loose flywheel ring that had to be hit with a hammer every so often, this was the sole mechanical failure of the entire trip.

The preliminary planning was very thorough. The safari would take ten weeks. A daily schedule was drawn up, giving the time of arrival and departure for each stop. All arrangements for overnight accommodations were made well in advance of their departure. Spare parts were collected for anything that, in Dr. Williams' expert opinion, might break down. As for medical supplies: "We took enough to look after ourselves," Burkitt says, "and we used to joke with each other and say, after all, we ought to be pretty safe medically: we were three doctors, laden down with medical equipment, making a beeline from one hospital to the next. But I don't think we had to use any of the medicine."

The safari started on October 7, 1961. In ten weeks, exactly as they had planned, they covered ten thousand miles, journeyed through twelve countries, and visited fifty-seven hospitals.*

The route is given here: for the record, for those who enjoy armchair travel, and for those who enjoy the bark and growl of African place names. Some of the smaller villages may not be found in the average atlas, and some will be found only with difficulty—if at all—on the large-scale Shell or Michelin touring maps.

* A factor of considerable importance to Denis Burkitt was that the Director of Medical Services at Mulago Hospital, Dr. William Davis, graciously (and wisely) recognized the ten weeks not as leave but as a period of duty.

From Kampala, Burkitt and Ted Williams drove south down the west shore of Lake Victoria to Bukoba; then to Ndolage; then, picking up Cliff Nelson, to Kibondo. Then to Kasulu, where they turned west and made a loop around to Kigoma and Ujiji, the meeting place of Stanley and Livingstone on Lake Tanganyika.

They then drove down an utterly desolate, tsetse-infested part of Tanzania to Mpanda; next to Sumbawanga; then to Abercorn, in Zambia.

Here once again they turned westward in a loop that took them to Fort Rosebery and back to the main road at Kasama. They doubled back to Abercorn, and bore east and south to Karonga on Lake Malawi (Lake Nyasa on maps that are more than a few years old).

Then to Livingstonia; Fort Jameson; Lilongwe; and Blantyre, where Burkitt spoke at a meeting and performed some operations.

The next stage, south from Blantyre, was extremely difficult. They had planned to drive southwest to Salisbury, but this proved impossible: the Zambesi was too low and the ferry across it had stopped running. They then drove due south, mostly over dirt roads, to Dona Ana, where they put the stationwagon on a goods train and crossed the Zambesi over what was then the longest bridge in the world. They resumed driving, thought they were lost (because their map was wrong), tried in vain to find their direction by a compass, which none of them could read, tried to find their direction by the moon, which gave them no information because it was directly overhead, and continued to drive all night until by good luck rather than intent they reached Beira, on the coast.

After a rest they turned westward to Umtali; up to Salisbury; then south to Fort Victoria and the Zimbabwe ruins, which John Gunther describes as "among the most formidable and mysterious in the world." They continued south, over Breit Bridge into Rhodesia, then through the Kruger National Park to Lourenço Marques, and westward again to Johannesburg, where they were greeted by George Oettlé.

They returned over the Breit Bridge once more, to Bulawayo; east to Wankie and Livingstone; up to Lusaka, through Broken Hill to Kitwe; then northeast across Zambia through Mpika and on to Mbeya; then up to Itigi, in the midst of more desolation, where the car had to be loaded on to a train (booked six months ahead) because the road marked on the map does not actually exist; to Tabora, where the car was unloaded; then on to Kola Ndoto (beside the Williamson diamond mines), where Cliff Nelson was working; and then to Mwanza, on the south shore of Lake Victoria. By boat, then, to Kisumu; and, finally, through torrential rain and floods, to Kampala.

At Lilongwe and Beira they saw children suffering from the tumor; but in general the hospitals they visited received no more than two or three cases a year, and it was therefore unlikely that on a given day Burkitt would find a child undergoing treatment. Some hospitals, of course, reported a much higher incidence of the disease: one, in Malawi, had admitted five patients in the preceding six months, while another in Tanzania had admitted six patients in three months. A pathologist in Lourenço Marques, Dr. Prates, had seen no less than forty children with the disease in the past four years, and he had assembled a remarkable collection of plaster models of some of these children, cast for him by the curator of the city museum. "An unusual form of medical witness," Burkitt calls this collection, and he was fascinated by it.

Everywhere he went, Burkitt gave lectures, held con-

ferences with doctors, nurses, and medical assistants, explaining what had brought him so far and what he was seeking.
The principal purpose of the safari was not simply to visit
hospitals reporting the tumor but *to discover where each
patient was living when the tumor first manifested itself.*
The location of the hospital was of secondary importance: it
might be ten, twenty, forty miles away. "We got a great deal
of information from records," Burkitt says: "We were able to
examine case sheets and find out where patients came from;
and a doctor might tell us, *Yes, we have seen a number of
these cases and they all came from that valley down there.*"
And this was what Burkitt needed to know in order to establish the edge he was seeking: exactly where the tumor occurred. The safari was really a highly ambitious exercise in
geographic pathology.

Several theories to explain the peculiar incidence of the
tumor had already been put forward by various people. One
theory was that the tumor belt across equatorial Africa, and
the tail extending south, corresponded to areas of radioactivity. Another theory suggested that the tumor might be related to diet; and yet another theory implicated mineral
deposits, or a *lack* of mineral deposits—such as molybdenum.

As the old stationwagon trundled down to Johannesburg
a new idea emerged. The three men sitting together on the
front seat of the Jubilee had an advantage denied to most
scientists: time—long uninterrupted stretches of time, time to
think and time to talk. "We discussed things as we went
along," Burkitt says. "We were enjoying ourselves, and we'd
talk about all the things we'd seen. I don't know who thought
of it first, whether it was Cliff or Ted or me—although I
imagine that Ted and Cliff probably made a much bigger
contribution than I did—but we suddenly realized that we

weren't finding *an edge* to the belt. *We were finding an altitude barrier.*"

What they had found was this: the tumor might be common in a particular area but—depending upon the locality—it stopped at a certain altitude.

Near the equator the tumor stopped at about 5,000 feet. *No cases occurred above this height.*

In Malawi (then Nyasaland), farther away from the equator, the altitude barrier was at 3,000 feet. *No cases occurred above this height.*

In Swaziland, still farther away from the equator, the altitude barrier fell to only 1,000 feet. *No cases occurred above this height.*

It was a remarkable finding, based entirely on the long careful process of establishing precisely where the tumor occurred. It was also a puzzling finding: why should a malignant tumor of human beings be dependent on *the altitude* at which those human beings lived?

Later, Burkitt wrote about this discovery, "In retrospect, I realize that relating the tumor to altitude was the result of the unhurried discussions possible on road travel but denied to the air traveler. I would almost certainly have missed the point had I traveled alone."

Back in Kampala there was, again, great interest in this new development. A human malignant tumor, a deadly human cancer, dependent upon altitude? Nobody had ever heard of such a thing, or even suspected such a thing. The ten thousand-mile safari in the old Jubilee stationwagon had proven to be more than worthwhile. Denis Burkitt, Ted Williams, and Cliff Nelson had contributed something original to medical science.

Their discovery was then taken a stage further by another of Burkitt's friends and colleagues, Professor A. J. Haddow, Director of the East African Virus Research Institute at Entebbe.

Haddow looked at Burkitt's findings and put another interpretation upon them. True, there was an altitude barrier. True, no cases occurred above a certain height, depending on the distance from the equator. But when the various altitudes were checked against the pattern of climate, Haddow showed that the altitude barrier was in fact *a temperature barrier, and the tumor did not occur where the temperature fell below about 60° F.* Therefore, where the temperature commonly fell below 60° F, children were unlikely to develop this tumor; where the temperature was commonly above 60° F the tumor was likely to occur. And this explained the strange business of altitude, for, obviously, the nearer you were to the equator the higher you had to go to reach the tumor-free zones where the temperature dropped below 60° F. Conversely, tumor-free areas, with a temperature below 60° F, were found at lower and lower altitudes the farther you traveled from the equator.

The excitement of discovery still ran high—perhaps even higher. Never before had a malignant tumor of human beings been related to climatic temperature. It was a milestone in geographic pathology.

"When we had reached that point," Burkitt says, "with such encouraging results, I felt a little more daring; and I asked if I could look around a little further. In fact, I asked if I could go to West Africa and see what was happening there. This was a short trip. I was there for only three weeks."

The same preliminary work had been done, of course:

mission and government hospitals had received Burkitt's questionnaires, letters had passed to and fro. And once more his characteristic method of investigation produced some striking and mysterious findings.

The tumor was common in the southern part of Nigeria.

But around Kano, a heavily populated area five hundred miles from Lagos, the tumor was exceedingly rare.

Something of the same sort happened in neighboring Ghana. The tumor could be found everywhere, except around Accra, on the coast.

And again Alex Haddow was able to provide an explanation.

This time the governing factor was rainfall. Government maps and statistical tables showed that in southern Nigeria and Ghana the annual rainfall is from 200 to 400 inches.

Kano, however, is close to the Sahara Desert, and it is in a local dry area (called by climatologists a rain shadow) with no more than 10 to 20 inches of rain a year.

Similarly, Accra is the driest part of the African coast, with an annual rainfall that is almost negligible.

The tumor had now been found to be dependent upon two factors: temperature and rainfall. It was a very unusual tumor indeed.

As a scientist one still had to be cautious. One could not, merely on the basis of two safaris, leap to conclusions. Some great matters were at stake here—insights, perhaps, into the mysteries of other forms of cancer.

So a third safari was planned, to the Republic of Rwanda; and for a number of reasons Burkitt's findings in Rwanda could be expected to settle the issues, one way or another.

Rwanda is one of the world's newest nations: until 1962

it was part of a sort of duplex nation, Rwanda-Urundi, under UN trusteeship administered by Belgium. It is approximately the size of Maryland, or Haiti, and it is the most densely populated country in Africa. It lies to the southwest of Uganda: the Republic of the Congo is to its west, and on the south is Burundi, which to the confusion of many Europeans was formerly Urundi. The Nile is considered to rise in the headwaters of Kagera River, which flows into Lake Victoria; and Rwanda is famous, additionally, for its giant Batusi (or Watusi), some of whom are more than seven and a half feet tall, and—at the other end of the human scale—its Batwa (or pygmies), most of whom are between four and five feet tall.

Essentially, Rwanda is a high plateau bristling with mountains, and with a great many beautiful lakes. John Gunther describes the road from Kisenyi to the capital, Astera (now Kigali), as "the most spectacular and dangerous I have ever traveled on." Lake Kivu, which forms part of the western border with the Congo, is typical of the region: it is 4,790 feet above sea level, and crocodiles (so the people living on the lakeshore say) cannot survive because the water is several degrees too cold for them.

In this high, heavily populated area, Burkitt could find no evidence of the tumor; no hospitals had seen it. Furthermore, many of the hospitals made a practice of sending specimens of tumor tissue to Mulago Hospital for identification, and Burkitt's tumor had never been reported. It simply did not occur at this altitude, where the temperature consistently falls below 60° F.

The story was different at Bujumbura, the capital of Burundi, about 250 miles from the equator on the extreme northeast corner of Lake Tanganyika. Bujumbura is comparatively low. Its altitude is only 2,625 feet and its climate is

D

hot and humid. Here, sure enough, the tumor was found to occur. The pattern held good: Rwanda and Bujumbura, for all intents and purposes, clinched the argument.

We make use of maps of many different kinds: maps showing the physical features of some particular territory—its shape, its national boundaries, its cities and villages, its mountains and its lakes and its rivers; maps showing geological data, or population patterns, or vegetation, or mineral deposits; maps showing the incidence of various forms of disease.

The map in Burkitt's office, dotted with hand-painted drawing pins, summarized all the evidence he had gathered in East Africa, West Africa, Rwanda, and finally Bujumbura.

Professor Haddow could provide a similar map, but by different means. Burkitt describes how he did it: "Alex looked at my map and said to himself, *What must I do to Africa to get a map like that?* And he found that if he rubbed chalk all over a map of Africa and then wiped off those areas where the rainfall was below 30 inches and the temperature fell below 60° F, he was left with an almost exact duplicate of my tumor map, simply on these factors of temperature and rainfall." This, of course, corresponded to the findings so far.

But Haddow went a step further. He asked himself, *What other map of Africa would have a similar pattern, with such emphasis on the factors of temperature and rainfall?* The answer was (and it came fairly easily to Professor Haddow because he is an entomologist): *an insect map of Africa.*

As luck would have it, Burkitt and Haddow were unable to lay their hands on a map of African mosquitoes, but in an old book on tsetse flies they found a map which fitted Burkitt's tumor map almost exactly. This did not implicate the tsetse fly because in many regions it had been wiped out since the book was printed: the map merely served to demonstrate that one insect, at least, could be related to those factors of rainfall and temperature associated with the tumor.

So there was now a *hint*, a *possibility*, that the tumor might be related to some insect. One had to be exceedingly cautious when one expressed this idea because nothing had been proven. Burkitt and Haddow only had a *suspicion* of a relationship, nothing more.

But another piece of evidence was added to the jigsaw puzzle as the result of the outbreak in 1959 of a disease called o'nyong nyong fever. This epidemic was, indeed, so severe that it has found a place in medical history, like the great influenza epidemics of 1918 and 1957. The disease causes the patient to feel that all his bones are broken (it is similar to dandy or breakbone fever), but it is rarely fatal.

Burkitt has given a vivid description of the epidemic: "It started in northwest Uganda. It raged across northern Uganda, affecting 98 percent of the population, *but when it reached an altitude of 5,000 feet it stopped.* It went around Lake Victoria. It went into part of southern Uganda. It went into Tanganyika. And everywhere it seemed to stop at about the same level as the tumor."

What is most interesting about o'nyong nyong fever is that it is caused by a virus; and this virus is carried by a mosquito. Professor J. N. P. Davies had already pointed out to Burkitt that his tumor map resembled a yellow fever map; and yellow fever, too, is caused by a virus carried by a mosquito. And at temperatures below 60° F the yellow fever viruses are unable to replicate themselves.

Nobody dared to say that Burkitt's tumor was actually

caused by a virus carried by mosquitoes.* Conclusive evidence was lacking. The circumstantial evidence, though, was enough to arouse excitement not only in Kampala but all over the world.

So Mr. Burkitt and his good friends and colleagues, working with research grants amounting to £275, riding around in an ancient Ford Jubilee stationwagon, seemed to have hit some kind of a jackpot. Here, for the first time, was a form of cancer that had every appearance of being related to an infection. "Once this thing got going," Burkitt says, "it went like a bombshell. I often say to people that if a boy goes on a picnic, and boils an egg, and by mistake sets fire to the prairie, you don't scold him, because he only meant to boil an egg. I am rather like that boy, only the fire went in a different way, and I really don't deserve any more credit than the boy deserves blame. But the fire went up. And it went up very quickly."

* Scientists prefer to use the term "arthropod." The arthropods include the *crustaceans* (lobsters, crayfish, crabs, shrimps, water fleas, and barnacles), the *arachnids* (spiders, scorpions, ticks, and mites), and *insects*, which are the largest class of all. Certain viruses carried by arthropods are called arboviruses, a piece of scientific shorthand derived from "*arthropod-borne*."

Interlude: You Cross
the Nile at Pakwach

One of the most significant clues to Denis Burkitt's character is his capacity for friendship. In the course of conversation he refers to his friends constantly, with great pride and with great affection. Many of them, of course, are in some branch of medicine; many of them share his religious beliefs; many of them have shared his African experience. "We have a full house," he wrote in a recent letter, "more than our six bedrooms can hold. We are often like this, and we give thanks that we have a home to which folks can come." In little more than two years, six hundred of his friends came to visit, by invitation or, as he says, "by just turning up."

Dr. E. H. Williams, chief engineer on the great tumor safari, belongs to the large group of men and women whom Burkitt refers to, broadly, as his best friends. The two men first met in 1948, but Ted Williams had encountered various members of the Burkitt family much earlier.

"I was born in Nairobi," he explains. "My father was in the Civil Service, and he was a personal friend of Denis's Uncle Roland—the first practicing surgeon in East Africa and a very remarkable man. I grew up with William Burkitt, the son of the great Dr. Burkitt (as we used to call him), and I remember the doctor saying in my presence, when I was a boy, that the Burkitts could trace their ancestry back to the Norman invasion of Ireland. They are very strong characters, these Burkitts."

The same can be said of the Williams family. Very strong characters. Very remarkable men.

Kuluva Hospital, where Dr. Ted Williams and Dr. Peter Williams live with their families, is about eight miles from the little township of Arua, in northwest Uganda. It is so far to the north that it is close to the border of Uganda and the Sudan, and so far to the west that it is very close to the border of Uganda and the Congo. It is remote, very remote. Many maps show Arua simply as a dot, with no roads leading to it; but this has changed. There are roads now, bumpy but passable.

The easiest way to reach Kuluva Hospital is to rent a plane in Kampala and fly the three hundred miles to Arua. That, however, is a costly way to travel, and it is more sensible to rent a car. It is still more sensible to engage a driver with your rented car, for even in fair weather the roads are treacherous and you are likely to encounter some unexpected hazards.

Your first stop will be at Masindi, 130 miles from Kampala, where there is a fine old colonial hotel with broad verandas and well-kept grounds, and where you can enjoy a cup of exceptionally good Ugandan coffee. Linger and savor the brew, because the opportunity will not occur again. Then you drive north to the Murchison Falls National Park, and if you are new to Africa you must turn off to see the Falls. They are magnificent. At this point the Victoria Nile is constricted from about half a mile in width to a few yards, and the wild, foaming water then plunges about a hundred and fifty feet and pours on—full of crocodiles, and giant perch weighing a hundred pounds or more, and bilharzia—to enter Lake Albert at Fort Magungo.

Your second stop will be at Paraa Lodge, which is usually crowded beyond its capacity and where you may have to wait an hour or so for a rather indifferent sandwich and a bottle of soapy Ugandan beer. Elephant and hippo come right up to the lodge, and you are warned, a little ironically, not to feed them. But you would be unwise to skip Paraa because it, and Masindi, are the only hotels on your route: you have no other choice.

Murchison Falls National Park is vast—miles and miles and miles of boring scrub. There seem to be great numbers of elephants, and since the park is not fenced in you will see herds of them outside the park boundaries. To someone who is not elephant-obsessed they appear to be brooding, malevolent, mountainous gray hulks, inhabiting a world of their own. In a herd they look like a slightly animated Stonehenge. They require, as an item of diet, a mineral contained in the bark of the local trees, and you drive through extensive areas of the park which look as if they have been devastated by ceaseless bombardment: every tree has been stripped of its bark by the elephants, every tree is grotesquely dead, every branch is gaunt, yellow, leafless, and the scene is one of utter desolation. If you are a student of ecology or a subscriber to the *New Statesman* you might immediately assume that this is another tragic example of the way man rapes and ruins his environment; but, no. Nature has been

raped and ruined here by her own pet pipe-nosed pachy-
derms.

At certain times of the year, too, you will drive through a
succession of bush fires, set by the game wardens in order to
burn off the old sour grass and bring up new grass, which
will attract the park animals so that they can be seen and ad-
mired by tourists. It is an eerie experience, driving into a
dense cloud of black smoke and crackling flame and coming
out upon a screeching assembly of birds—huge marabou
storks, demoiselle cranes, kites, even secretary birds, picking
off the insects and small animals fleeing the fire. Scavengers.
They resent you, and you soon learn to resent them.

When you leave the northern gate of the park you enter
tsetse fly territory (and on your return trip some lackadaisi-
cal guards will flick the inside of your car with long whisks
to make sure you have not acquired any of these pestiferous
creatures, the carriers of sleeping sickness). Now you will see
herdsmen riding bicycles and carrying nine-foot spears, terribly dangerous weapons with a broad spearhead at one end
and a long, sharp spike at the other end; and if you ask your
driver why the men carry these things he will tell you, "To
defend themselves." "To defend themselves against what?"
"Their enemies," the driver will say; but he may then admit
that the spears are to kill any game that strays out of the
park. It is forbidden, but the people have a desperate need
for meat, and there are not enough game wardens to stop the
poaching. So, day by day and night by night, the animals
mysteriously vanish.

You cross the Nile at Pakwach. This is the Albert Nile,
flowing out of Lake Albert, but indistinguishable from any
other stretch of that ancient river. Chances are good that the
ferry will have broken down, and you will have to wait patiently while repairs are made. You will not be alone. There

will be a long line of trucks and safari cars, and there will be
scores of poor Africans waiting with you, some of them strid-
ing up and down and abusing the government in passionate
tones, because the government is supposed to be responsible
for running the ferries. The Nile is broad, fast-moving, and it
looks dirty, perhaps because it carries a great deal of mud,
as well as sewage; and you are likely to be distressed by the
Africans' general indifference to self-preservation—they wade
into the dirty brown water, splash it over themselves to cool
off, drink cupped handfuls of it, give it to their children to
drink. You can understand why they suffer from a multiplic-
ity of frightful diseases; the mystery is how any of them
manage to survive.

Once across the river you are in the West Nile District of
Uganda, which stretches—as its name implies—from the west
bank of the Nile to the Congo border (on the west) and to
the Sudan (on the north). It is a single government administrative unit, according to Dr. Williams, with a population
of about half a million comprising four main tribes, and its
area is slightly less than that of Wales. The scenery is a
welcome change from the flat scrub of the national park: it
is rather like the more picturesque sections of the Rhine Valley—lush and wooded, with sugarloaf mountains rising in the
distance. Your driver will put on speed now, because he is
uneasy in this territory on the other side of the Nile. He is
among alien people whose language he cannot understand
and who regard him with suspicion. From Pakwach it is some
eighty miles to Kuluva Hospital, and despite the condition of
the red-mud road he will cover the distance in less than an
hour and a half. He will be unaware that this district has won
a place in medical history, and at the back of his mind he
will undoubtedly be asking himself why on earth you had to

D*

come to such a forsaken spot. Not Godforsaken. It is far from that.

Most of us exist within a small circle from which we rarely escape: certain rooms in a certain building in a certain street in a certain country. We may move from one place to another, but the change is usually insignificant. We do certain kinds of work and society rewards us with certain benefits: we have hot and cold running water and efficient disposal systems; we can obtain a variety of foods without having to carry nine-foot spears all the time; we are provided with numerous pleasures and luxuries—films, theaters, concerts, books, fine clothes, speedy automobiles; we have extensive medical facilities to care for our physical well-being, drugs to put us to sleep and drugs to wake us up. But at some time or another most of us become conscious of the smallness of our own particular circle, we are alarmed by its limitations, and we ask ourselves if this is why we were granted the miracle of life, merely to exist within such a tiny enclosure, devoid of any important challenge, devoid of spiritual or physical joy, devoid of adventure, devoid of beliefs. We wonder: What would it be like to break out of the little circle, to do work (unspecified) that will test all our muscles, to deny ourselves the enfeebling benefits and pleasures that society provides? Then, after agonizing over this prospect for a while, after some juvenile tantrums because Fate has treated us so badly, the circle quietly encloses us again and life goes on in the old settled way. We rarely escape. The traffic lights are *all* red; they remain red; and if they ever turned to green few of us would know what to do next.

The Kuluva story begins with a God-fearing wine merchant in the City of London, Mr. Hammond, who endowed several beds in the London Hospital (and made a practice of visiting them every Sunday afternoon to comfort the occupants). Among other good deeds, he became a godfather to Edward Hammond Williams and left him a legacy that helped to pay for the young man's medical education at St. Bartholomew's Hospital. Dr. Williams then went to the Mildmay Mission Hospital in the East End of London to complete his internship; here he met a nurse named Muriel Edith Mary Francis, whom he married.

In 1941 they sailed from England to Africa to begin life as missionaries. They were fortunate to arrive: the ship taking them to Cape Town narrowly missed being torpedoed by a Nazi submarine.

After three months of traveling, Ted and Muriel Williams boarded a paddle steamer on the Albert Nile and chugged upstream to Rhino Camp, in those days "a meagre collection of buildings, partly for the benefit of the East African Railways & Harbours and partly connected with a Cotton Ginnery," now a tourist landmark. They were met by two missionaries in a car named *The Yellow Peril* and driven to Arua, forty miles due west, the main mission station for the district.*

No *medical* missionaries had worked here up to this time. Dr. Williams and his wife began the venture with the barest

---

* Nobody can tell this story better than Dr. Williams himself, and much of this account is taken from a booklet written by him entitled "Probably *Not:* The Story of Kuluva," published by the Africa Inland Mission, 3 John Street, London, W.C.1, price 6d (about 6¢); unfortunately out of print. Here once more we encounter aspects of personal faith not too frequently found in descriptions of scientific discovery and accomplishment; but any reader whose chief concern is scientific enlightenment need not worry: there is plenty ahead.

minimum of equipment plus about £10 (then about $50) in funds.

"God sent a tremendous test to the faith of the two missionaries," writes Dr. Williams. "No gifts arrived to supplement the £10 capital and the meagre equipment already in hand. For three months the heavens seemed as brass, and the Faith Basis of the Mission meaningless. Nevertheless, a start was made. Two dilapidated one-room buildings were repaired, and fittings manufactured from packing cases. It seemed queer doing operations under a bare thatched roof with no protective ceiling. . . . In their home the two missionaries did not find things very thrilling: there was no glass in the windows, just a bamboo lattice; bare whitewashed walls, dusty floor, lots of white ants attacking suitcases and furniture nightly. . . . Then quite suddenly the Lord sent £50 for a car, and £300 for buildings, and other gifts which enabled much needed medical supplies to be ordered. An old car was bought for £27 10s [$137], some necessary spare parts purchased with the balance of the original gift; and this car did yeoman service for seven and a half years. . . . The element of doubt loomed large in the minds of the two missionaries. Outside observers, if asked if this venture would ever succeed, would no doubt have replied, 'Probably not.' Surely, the call, guiding and purpose seemed mistaken. Something was wrong somewhere."

What was wrong, perhaps, was human frailty: the lack of a few material things, such as money and equipment. But the first year passed, "and with it came the dawn of a new comprehension of the opportunity and challenge of the work. Soon a few small buildings were built. The doctor's wife would look after the bulk of the patients each morning, leaving a few for her husband to see in moments snatched from building operations. The afternoons were mostly spent in making window frames and hospital furniture.

"These," Dr. Williams says, "were busy and fruitful years, but not years of real expansion in the work. God's time for this had not yet come, though much was being learned, such as language, customs, people, building, car mechanics and a host of smaller things." Two daughters were born, Joy and Mollie, and Dr. Williams relates how one of them, only four years old, "slipped unnoticed into the operating theatre one day when an emergency operation for the amputation of a leg, to save the life of a little boy, was being performed. The atmosphere was tense, for it was touch and go. While the doctor's wife concentrated on giving the anesthetic, the doctor wielded knife and surgical saw with all speed, and the little girl's presence passed unnoticed until the amputation was completed. Then with a shock she was noticed. But she was merely sorry for the little boy and quite unmoved by an operation which would make the average adult go into a faint. Later, when it came to teaching the little boy to walk on crutches, the missionaries' child learned first, and then moved by her sympathy for the little boy's plight, she taught him herself."

After World War II, interest in the problem of leprosy in Africa (and elsewhere) grew considerably. Surveys showed unsuspected concentrations of leprosy victims, but at the same time the development of new drugs provided more effective treatment of the disease, which is caused by a microorganism similar to the tuberculosis bacillus.

"God also guided in the enlargement of the existing medical work in the West Nile to include leprosy, but this could not be attempted on the already overcrowded Arua station site. . . . One day a friendly chief was taken for a drive to look for a possible new site in the area under his jurisdiction. As the car was driven along a well-known stretch of land, an area of land on the right of the road suddenly seemed to take on a new significance. It was dominated by a hill, a well-known landmark, called Kuluva. Years later, piecing together the meaning of this name—"a place of strife"—and fragments of history, it seems clear that long ago a clan lived in this place who may have been from a tribe of iron-workers. Fragments of slag, the remains of an old hearth, and a primitive stone tool have been found to support this supposition. It appears that this clan, by its cruel and frequent raids on the clans around, earned their bitter hatred until one day they banded together and massacred the iron-workers. Since that time, the land had remained uninhabited, yet ready in the purpose of God for the Africa Inland Mission to occupy it decades later.

"Lease formalities for 200 acres took about a year to complete, and then one day beside the road thirty workmen were engaged to start developing the land. A road was begun, boundaries were demarcated, and work was started on a plantation of eucalyptus trees.

"It took five years to build Kuluva and develop its work. This is fairly rapid growth in Africa Inland Missionary history and is a wonderful indication of the Lord's provision and guidance. Building with bricks, mud mortar, eucalyptus poles and grass . . . between forty and fifty brick buildings, inexpensive and therefore not of too high a quality or degree of permanence, have been erected, using perhaps half a million bricks. . . .

"So bit by bit the work enlarged from the original thirty leprosy patients to a total of 350; from twelve hospital beds to forty; from 30,000 outpatient attendances a year to 70,000."

❅   ❅   ❅

This was written by Dr. Williams in 1955, fourteen years after he and his wife stepped off the paddle steamer at Rhino Camp, with £10 in funds and a minimum of medical equipment.

The friendly chief who led them to Kuluva had driven south with them from Arua. Approached from this direction the "place of strife" was on the right. You, driving north from Kampala, will see the site on your left; and entering the hospital grounds by a sweeping semicircle of rough road, you will find that those two untried and inexperienced young missionaries have accomplished wonders. Kuluva is a miracle. Ted Williams has now lost count of the number of buildings he and his African workmen (recruited from neighboring villages) have erected: between fifty and sixty, he will tell you, or perhaps more. Various people have come to Kuluva to help: his brother Peter, also a doctor, specializing in ophthalmology, arrived in 1948. Soon after they were joined by their parents.*

* Dr. Williams writes, in a personal communication: "Our present staff at Kuluva consists of the following: Fourteen Ugandan dressers trained at Kuluva, two record clerks, and other ancillary workers, totaling about forty. There are two expatriate (non-Ugandan) doctors, brothers, and their wives, both registered nurses and midwives; three nursing sisters (the title given if they are both nurses and midwives), expatriate, for the hospital, two nursing sisters for the leprosy work, and one sister with special training in ophthalmology—my brother, of course, being trained in this specialty (we see a great deal of onchocerciasis). We also have an expatriate manager, and his wife, who does the accounts.

We have had perhaps 35 to 40 medical students here in the last nine years from England and America, of which perhaps a dozen have been Smith Kline and French Fellowship students. They seem to find the experience here stimulating and very worthwhile."

Every morning, before lunch, Dr. and Mrs. Williams see, on an average, some three hundred outpatients, and in the afternoons Dr. Ted performs operations. In the evenings, whenever necessary, he drives out to the villages to see those who are unable to leave their homes. Kuluva Hospital is the nearest hospital of any kind for twenty thousand people in the West Nile District. It has seventy-five beds today, and in part—but only in part—the problem of nursing is solved by having relatives come in to look after patients. In the past ten years Ted Williams has treated *seven thousand* leprosy patients, and two hundred and fifty live in villages all through the valley.

"We have always tried to have better equipment than buildings," he says. "A lot of the buildings are just sun-dried brick, and they should last about twenty years. Then we can pull them down and put up better buildings.

"But a major part of our job is to propagate our faith, and this is not a reason for practicing second-class medicine. We must practice absolutely first-class medicine; and with that goes the Christian message, which is all-important to us. Practicing first-class medicine today, though, isn't easy.

"Wherever you go in the world—even in an out-of-the-way place like this—the problems of hospitals are the problems of cost. Two-thirds of costs are wages, and we often wonder where mission hospitals will go in the future. Medical treatment gets more and more expensive. The equipment you need for tests gets more and more expensive. People who come out new to work here have no idea of economy— *what we mean by economy*. They're accustomed to all sorts of disposable things—disposable this, disposable that.

"Here, we use a disposable syringe for two months."

*   *   *

Ted Williams' decision to become a missionary doctor can be traced directly to a child's book about David Livingstone, given to him when he was six years old and still one of his most precious possessions. Half a century after Livingstone's death his words still had the power to inspire boys and men to seek out the most inaccessible places in Africa, to bring light and hope into darkness. *Do you carry on the work I have begun. I leave it with you.*

What helped to make Ted Williams one of the leading figures in the Burkitt story can also be traced back to his boyhood: a passion for maps, acquired from his father, who was Chief Computer in the Kenya Survey Department, a title that denoted he was in charge of the mapping section. Many years later, stimulated by Denis Burkitt during the great tumor safari, Dr. Williams began to plot on large-scale maps all cases of Burkitt's lymphoma (and other malignancies, such as cancer of the liver) he encountered at Kuluva Hospital.

Obviously, if he only plotted where the disease was first reported, it would appear that all cases had occurred at the hospital itself (and absurd as it seems, this is the way statistics are assembled in some areas). The key factor is *where the child lived when he or she showed the first signs of the disease.* "It's easy for me," Dr. Williams says. "With every one of my cases, after I've treated the child I take him, or her, home myself. So I know exactly where that child came from. And this *detailed plotting* is of tremendous importance. It is something that should be done by all missionary doctors who live and work for a lengthy period in underdeveloped countries."

The reason is that virtually all underdeveloped countries are now in process of development. In most parts of Africa the pattern of life is changing with extraordinary speed. Until recently, for example, the population of a fairly remote region like the West Nile District was relatively stable. Few people ever traveled more than a few miles from the village where they were born, simply because the means for travel were unavailable. Even a cheap bicycle was far beyond the means of the average man.

Now there is a daily bus to Kampala, and it has been estimated that about thirty thousand West Nilers travel to Kampala every year. Furthermore, the government is building a magnificent bridge across the Nile at Pakwach, to carry a railroad as well as cars and bicycles and pedestrians, and the old, inefficient ferry will soon be forgotten. People will move freely from place to place in Uganda, as they do anywhere else in the world; and as a consequence, keeping track of any disease will become increasingly difficult.

"We have perhaps ten years left here in which to do the detailed mapping of cases of cancer," Ted Williams explains. "I don't know the precise significance of my plotting. But we can say with certainty that *there*, on that spot on the map, a case of some particular kind of cancer occurred. And some indication of the value of this work is that the East African Virus Research Institute is making a copy of every one of my maps, so that there will be two records in existence."

By pure luck he works in a district which has an unusually high incidence of Burkitt's lymphoma: two to four times higher than elsewhere in Uganda, and higher, possibly, than anywhere in the world. It is not lucky that so many West Nile children develop the disease; it *is* lucky, and perhaps providential, that Dr. Williams happens to be there and can do something useful about the disease—treating its victims and helping to find the means to put an end to it. And his observations, his thinking, the evidence of his maps, have attracted scores of cancer scientists to Kuluva. "There is a tremendous concentration of scientists in this district at the moment," he said at the end of December 1968. "Investigators from the (British) Imperial Cancer Research Fund have come up four times this year, and they've carried out biological surveys on six hundred children. The Director of the East African Virus Research Institute, Dr. G. W. Kafuko, has been up here five times this year doing malaria surveys. Entomologists from the Institute came once a month to supervise mosquito catching: for two years they caught mosquitoes every single night in different parts of the district, and up to the end of last year they did special mosquito catches at every single home where Burkitt's lymphoma has occurred. These mosquitoes were sent back on ice; they were typed (that is, classified); and they were then ground up and examined for viruses. We don't have anything very dramatic yet, but we've established a pattern of viruses that are carried by mosquitoes, and you can draw a map of the West Nile showing these factors."

The maps display other factors, too. South of Arua there is a large area which is of great interest because no cases of Burkitt's lymphoma have occurred in it—a so-called "negative" or "blank" area. "In this blank area of ours," says Dr. Williams, "there are hardly any cattle. Up north, where most cases of the tumor occur, there are lots of cattle."

"Or, again, in the blank area there are no eucalyptus trees. In the tumor area up north there are lots of eucalyptus trees.

"Or, another curious thing: I've mapped the way tobacco cultivation has increased in this district. The tobacco plant, as everybody knows, harbors certain viruses. And it's very interesting that there is an almost 100 percent correlation between where Burkitt's tumor has occurred in the last sixteen or seventeen years, and how it has widened out, and how tobacco cultivation has widened out.

"Then there's the charnockite theory. Charnockite is a peculiar kind of rock, and if you plot charnockite formations on a map and compare them with the occurrence of Burkitt's tumor, there is a similarity: so much so that the information has been sent to London for computer analysis. It may turn out to be a factor.

"None of these things, so far, mean anything in themselves. But one day they may provide an important clue, and I just keep my eyes open for them, that's all."

The first time Ted Williams saw a child suffering from Burkitt's tumor was in 1942, one year after he and his wife arrived in Arua. He took photographs and—like Denis Burkitt fifteen years later—found himself puzzled by the child's condition. He continued to see cases of the disease year after year, and they continued to puzzle him. "I can show you some notes I made on a case in 1953: I couldn't make out why the child had a tumor of its orbit (the eye socket) and a tumor of the abdomen. On another card, my brother has written, *What IS this peculiar cancer?* We sent tissue specimens to the laboratories, and they couldn't help us."

This was a period, in Ted Williams' opinion, when cancer research found itself in a blind alley. "Researchers were reading papers *to* each other, writing papers *for* each other, and getting nowhere.

"Then Denis Burkitt came along. The great thing about Denis was that first and foremost he was a clinician, actually working with patients in a hospital. He broke out of the normal pattern of research (which is generally carried on in a laboratory) by observing *as a clinician* a tumor occurring in several sites in children. He went outside the laboratory, again, to track this tumor down, to find where and how it occurred; then he passed this information on to the laboratory researchers so that they could define what the tumor was.

"What he did, in fact, was to alter the whole concept of research. He showed that the clinicians, particularly people who work for a long time in one place—as we missionaries do—are in a position to assemble a great deal of unique and extremely valuable information.

"I can say this for myself: For years, research was something one read about in scientific journals. It required a lot of expensive equipment, and one never thought that one could start any kind of useful research in a remote place like this. It was Denis Burkitt who put me (and many other people in similar situations) on to the idea that *the research material is right here where we're working.*"

Ted and Muriel Williams live in a sort of bungalow—the last building to be completed in their building program. The living room is large and low and comfortable, and filled with the warmth of the people who live in it. Dr. Ted sits in an old armchair, surrounded by books and papers and maps and photographs, and he is perfectly willing to talk to you half the night, until his voice cracks with tiredness.

He cannot predict the future of Kuluva Hospital, or even his own future. Eventually, he tells you, all medical services in Uganda will be nationalized, and it is probable that Kuluva will be taken over by the government. "We should realize that we may not be here in ten years' time in our present form. We get some money from the government now, but we often wonder when it will stop. The Ugandans, perhaps rightly, feel we shouldn't be earning money that should go to Ugandans."

Meanwhile the work goes on: the healing and comforting of the sick, the promulgation of faith, the various research projects, the maps, the endless asking of questions. And the great tumor safari is very fresh in his memory. He laughs in wonderment as he recalls it. "The total cost of that piece of research work," he says, "including buying the car, having it thoroughly overhauled before we started on the trip, then selling it for a lower price afterwards; including our meals and staying at rest houses (and, to our consternation, staying at the best hotel in Johannesburg when we arrived there because our friends had booked us into it); *the total cost* of that trip was £650.

"At the time it was about two thousand dollars; and that's what Smith Kline and French give one student on a fellowship to come here for ten weeks. There were three of us on that safari; and I would think that at £650 it's the cheapest piece of major research of this century."

10

Bombshell

We have to bear in mind that Uganda is, after all, a relatively small country. Its capital, Kampala, is a relatively small city, not very well known outside Africa. Mulago Hospital is the teaching hospital of East Africa and thus an exceedingly important institution, but few medical men in Europe or America are aware of its importance or even of its existence.

So it seems improbable that the scientific world would be wildly excited by the news that one of the surgeons—the third in order of seniority, to be precise—in distant Mulago Hospital, in Darkest Africa, had come upon an unusual tumor affecting only a few hundred children a year. True, as Burkitt said, "Once this thing got going it went like a bombshell"; the miracle is that the news actually reached the outside world, that there was an opportunity for it to *get going*, instead of being totally ignored, as so often happens. One thinks of the Abbé Mendel, working patiently in his monastery garden in Brünn: his Laws of inheritance were published in 1866 and 1869, and went unnoticed until they were discovered by the Dutch botanist De Vries in 1900. Or, on another order, one thinks of Alexander Fleming, who in 1928 discovered penicillin by a chance observation (it happened to be the chance observation of a genius) and then had to wait ten years for further investigation of his findings.

Scientists do not deliberately ignore each other's work. There is no conspiracy to prevent the spread of medical knowledge. The problem is simple: such a torrent of scientific papers pours out of medical centers all over the world that it is utterly impossible for any human being to keep up with what is going on even in his own special field. Unless a discovery is of obvious importance, the likelihood is that it will pass unnoticed. Or it may attract attention briefly and then disappear in the deluge of the next day's papers.

It is interesting, consequently, to see with what generosity Providence treated Denis Burkitt.

He first discussed the tumor informally, without a paper, at one of the Saturday morning staff meetings in Mulago Hospital.

"I first presented it *officially*," he says, "at the annual meeting of the East African Association of Surgeons, in January 1958, at Kampala."

The emphasis here is on *surgeons*, and this becomes more apparent in the next stage of the story, for Burkitt's first published article on the tumor was in the *British Journal of Surgery*, in 1959. "I wanted to publish in a surgical journal because I was a surgeon," he explains, "although some of my colleagues said I should have published in a journal of pathology." For once his colleagues were right and he was wrong.

"It was received with a complete lack of interest. It didn't strike a bell with anybody." *

The next paper was written in collaboration with J. N. P. Davies, Professor of Pathology at Makerere University College Medical School. It was published in 1961. If the first paper was printed in a surgical journal because Mr. Burkitt was a surgeon, one can predict with a fair degree of certainty where he would wish the second paper to be printed; and one would be absolutely right. It appeared in an Irish journal called the *Medical Press,* which had asked Burkitt for a contribution. "This paper," he says with a bright Irish smile, "created a *little* interest."

The third paper was written by Burkitt and Dr. G. T. O'Conor, another member of the Department of Pathology at Makerere. It, too, appeared in 1961, but this time Burkitt was on the right track. He chose the periodical *Cancer,* published in Philadelphia, which is read by cancer experts not only in the United States but internationally. The same issue carried another article about the lymphoma, written by Dr. O'Conor; and it was these two articles that really sparked interest in Burkitt's work. "After these papers came out," he says, "people said, *This is something.* There were leaders in *The New York Times,* and so on; and we were flooded with requests for reprints."

* Medical readers may like to know of Burkitt's other papers. They are given here with his comments: "A Simple Serviceable Artificial Leg" (*E. A. Med. J.,* 1953). *This is still being made sixteen years later.* "A Boot and Caliper Bank" (*E. A. Med. J.,* 1960). *This has been modified since.* "A Simple Crutch" (*B. Med. J.,* 1961). *This has been very rewarding and very widely used.* "Subcutaneous Phycomycosis" (with other authors: *B. Med. J.,* 1964). "Relics of Tradition" (*E. A. Med. J.,* 1965). *Very provocative.*

Altogether, a total of four papers, published in less than two years, made Burkitt's tumor known to cancer scientists all over the world.

And in this way the bombshell went off.

One can ask, Precisely why did the news of Burkitt's tumor produce such a strong reaction in the world community of cancer scientists? What, really, was so special, so significant, so unusual, about a disease that afflicts no more than a few hundred African children every year? What made Burkitt's tumor so much more exciting to cancer scientists than, say, cancer of the lung, which kills about sixty thousand people a year in the United States alone, or cancer of the stomach, which kills vast numbers of people in such widely separated countries as Japan and Chile and Finland and Austria?

The answers are remarkably interesting; but we have to arrive at them by a rather roundabout route. Some of the answers, indeed, can only be given when more of the Burkitt story has been told.

There is no need to stress the fact that cancer is a major problem of mankind. In most developed countries, where people have a span of life approaching the Biblical threescore years and ten, it is the second leading cause of death, after heart disease. We fear it because its effects are grim, and also because it seems to attack us without rhyme or reason (except where there is a clear relationship, as in cancer of the lung, which is for the most part directly associated with the smoking of cigarettes). At the time Burkitt began his investigations only one form of cancer, called choriocarcinoma, could be cured by means of drugs alone, in a certain percentage of cases. Other forms of the disease could be cured only by means of surgery or radiotherapy, when these techniques could be applied. In general, drugs were held to be palliative; they helped to suppress the disease, they helped to extend the patient's life, but they were not by themselves curative.

Cancer does not occur without rhyme or reason, of course. It is subject, like everything else, to the laws of nature, and although it has many mysterious aspects we can be fairly certain that sooner or later these mysteries will be solved. We cannot say when: perhaps within twenty-five years, perhaps not for two hundred and fifty years. If we can walk on the moon, if we can take close-up photographs of Mars, then we can learn what causes cells to behave abnormally. Meanwhile, every clue, every lead, is of value.

In effect the rational study of cancer began in 1915, when two Japanese scientists at the University of Tokyo, Professor K. Yamagiwa and Professor K. Ichikawa, were able to induce skin cancer in rabbits by dabbing the ears with coal tar. Dabbing the ears once, twice, a dozen times, was insufficient. The process had to be continued regularly for more than six months.

Fifteen years later, Sir Ernest Kennaway, working with several colleagues in London, found one of the substances in coal tar which causes skin cancer. Its name is uninspiring, but it is renowned in medical history: 3,4-benzpyrene.

The importance of these discoveries was that, for the first time, scientists had the means to study cancer in the laboratory. They could produce skin cancer in controlled tests on certain animals; they could follow the progress of skin cancer from the first tissue changes to the ultimate malignancy.

From this beginning, immense benefits have been won. We now know many causes of skin cancer—excessive exposure to sunlight is possibly the most serious; but, more significant than anything else, we have learned that cancer is not always an unmitigated disaster. In the United States some 110,000 cases of skin cancer are reported in a year. Of these, only about 5,000 will be fatal; 105,000 will be cured.

This high cure rate is easily explained. Skin cancer occurs on the outer surface of the body, where it is readily seen and can be effectively treated. The changes in the skin usually take place over a long period of time—as much as twenty to forty years—and they are not likely to be overlooked.

It would be wonderful if all cancers could be recognized as easily, and could be treated with the same degree of success. The obvious problem with cancers occurring below the surface of the body is that frequently they remain completely hidden from view: they do not even manifest themselves as a lump. The early changes take place "silently"—that is, they are painless and produce no symptoms; and in adults a malignancy may progress for a long time before it is diagnosed. Cancer of the stomach, for example, may take about twenty-five years to mature. A man may begin to smoke cigarettes at the age of sixteen, and cancer of the lung is not likely to manifest itself until he is in his forties. In certain other forms of cancer the induction time may be as long as fifty years.

The cancer researcher is thus faced with peculiar difficulties. Assume that he is investigating stomach cancer. The only effective treatment for this disease at present is surgery. *If we could learn what causes stomach cancer* we might then take steps to prevent it from occurring at all.

But how can the scientist go about the task of finding the cause of this particular malignancy? Where can he begin? First and foremost, he is faced with the fact that the disease matures very slowly, over a period of twenty-five years or so. He cannot *predict* that it will strike a certain person. He cannot *see* the early changes leading to the growth of the tumor. He is unable to acquire vital information about the individual's condition when these early changes began to occur—about diet, allergies, vitamin deficiencies, and a thousand and one other factors that might affect the malignant process.*

Probably the most perplexing of all forms of cancer are the lymphomas (which were described earlier) and leukemia.

The name "leukemia" means "white blood condition," and it is actually a generic term for a number of different kinds of cancer that for the most part affect the white blood cells. In the United States about fourteen thousand adults and children die of leukemia each year. One way of classifying the different forms is according to the length of time the patient lives after the disease is recognizable: *acute,* less than six months; *sub-acute,* up to about a year; *chronic,* more than a year.

Chronic leukemia is the form most common in adults. It develops very slowly, and may continue for three years or more. In some patients the disease can be controlled very well, and many cases have been reported of patients who have lived for ten years or more after their disease was first diagnosed.

Acute leukemia is the form most common in children, although it may also affect adults. Without treatment the course of the disease is often exceedingly rapid, but new

* This is purely a hypothetical example. Research has not been able to pinpoint the cause, or causes, of stomach cancer, but much has been learned about it indirectly. It is "associated" with diet—with an excessive intake of starchy foods such as rice or potatoes; it is also "associated" with an excessive intake of smoked foods. Other "associations" are pernicious anemia, vitamin A deficiency, and peptic ulcers. Obviously, research on stomach cancer is exceedingly difficult, and we may have to wait some time to learn how it is caused.

drugs and new techniques can now help to extend life very considerably.

In the past quarter of a century there has been a concentration of research on leukemia. Again and again, scientists appeared to be close to a cure for one form of the disease or another; again and again the hope has been frustrated. Most disappointing, leukemia in all its forms is still a total mystery. We know that it can arise from excessive exposure to radiation, and possibly from the action of certain chemicals, particularly benzene; but these can cause only a tiny fraction of all the cases of leukemia occurring throughout the world. We have to admit that the cause, or causes, of human leukemia are unknown; and yet there is widespread confidence today that we are close to finding *a cause*. The magic word is "viruses."

In 1908, fifty years before Denis Burkitt set off on his first tumor safari, two Danish scientists, Wilhelm Ellermann and Olaf Bang, transmitted leukemia from one chicken to another by injecting a fluid obtained by filtering blood and tissue that had been affected by the disease. The fluid contained no leukemic cells (and is therefore called a cell-free filtrate), and the scientists concluded that the "infectious agent" which passed from one chicken to the other in this fluid must be a virus.

There was little progress in leukemia-virus research for the next forty years. In 1951, Dr. Ludwik Gross of New York, following a lead provided by Dr. Gilbert Dalldorf, was able to induce leukemia in newborn mice by means of a cell-free filtrate obtained from mice suffering from leukemia. Again, the conditions of the experiment were such that the infectious agent could only be a virus.

Subsequently, researchers found more than two dozen

viruses related in some way to murine leukemia (that is, leukemia occurring in rats or mice, as distinct from avian leukemia, which occurs in fowl and other birds). Particles that have the *appearance* of viruses have been found in a variety of animals—cats, dogs, and cattle.

Scientists could now argue that since viruses cause certain kinds of leukemia in animals, there is a strong possibility that viruses might be the cause of certain kinds of leukemia in man; and, in fact, several scientists have reported seeing "virus particles" in human leukemic tissue examined with the electron microscope. But evidence of this sort is very difficult to assess. True, the viruses may be *in* the leukemic tissue. How can we prove, though, that these viruses *caused* the leukemia? The difficulty is that we cannot take these virus particles (even if we could obtain them in sufficient numbers) and inject them into human beings. If we attempted to do so, and if the virus particles actually caused leukemia in a human being, the experiment would be legally tantamount to murder, for to all intents and purposes acute leukemia is invariably fatal.

Burkitt and his colleagues supplied the breakthrough. Those two papers published in *Cancer* in 1961 must have seemed sensational to all scientists who had been working on the mystery of leukemia. There was still no absolute and final proof. Nothing was yet certain. But that remarkable company of men, Denis Burkitt and Ted Williams and Cliff Nelson and Jack Davies and Greg O'Conor, had come up with a human lymphoma which *appeared* to be dependent on certain factors of temperature and rainfall. From these findings arose the *suspicion* that some arthropod *might* be implicated as the carrier of an infectious agent which *played a part* in causing the disease; and the evidence *suggested* that the arthropod *might very well* be a mosquito; and that the infectious agent *might very well* be a virus.

Scientists, particularly cancer scientists, have to be exceedingly cautious. Unless the proof is absolutely indisputable they must guard any statement with multitudes of qualifying phrases. Nevertheless, there could be no mistaking the significance of Burkitt's tumor. If a virus seemed to be involved in this particular form of human lymphoma, a virus (but not necessarily the same virus) might be involved in some forms of human leukemia. And—to carry the thought a stage further, to its supreme conclusion—many diseases caused by viruses can be controlled by means of vaccines.

It was tremendous news, when its implications were understood. With very good reason, it exploded in scientific circles (as Mr. Burkitt said) like a bombshell; and there were more bombshells to come.

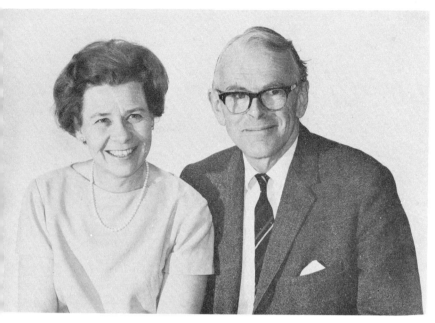

Denis and Olive Burkitt.

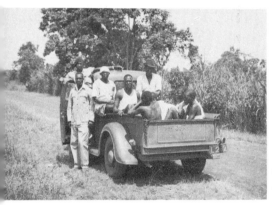

The old pick-up truck
taking patients to
Lira Hospital.

The operating theatre
in Lira Hospital.

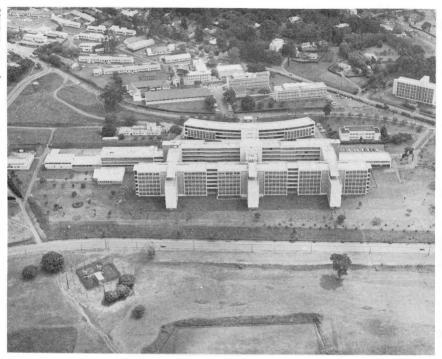

The magnificent new Mulago Hospital in Kampala, Uganda. The old Mulago Hospital is visible near the top left-hand corner.

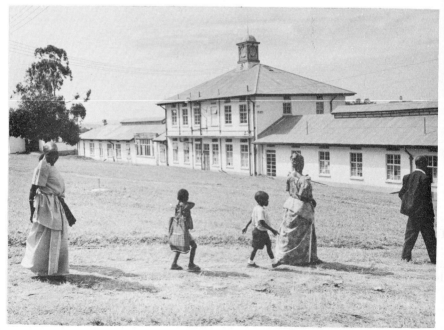

Old Mulago Hospital, Kampala.

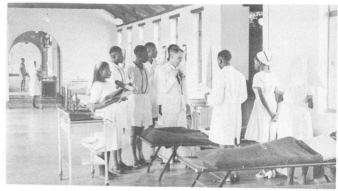

Dr. Hugh Trowell with some of his African medical students in the old Mulago Hospital. The photograph was taken in 1950.

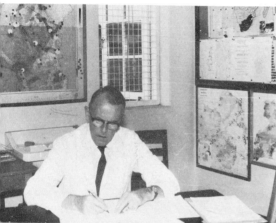

Denis Burkitt.

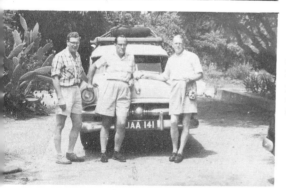

Dr. Clifford Nelson, Dr. E. H. Williams, and D. P. Burkitt at the start of the long safari.

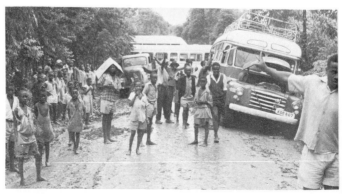

Torrential rains made roads virtually impassable on the last hundred miles of the long safari.

The "Lymphoma Belt"

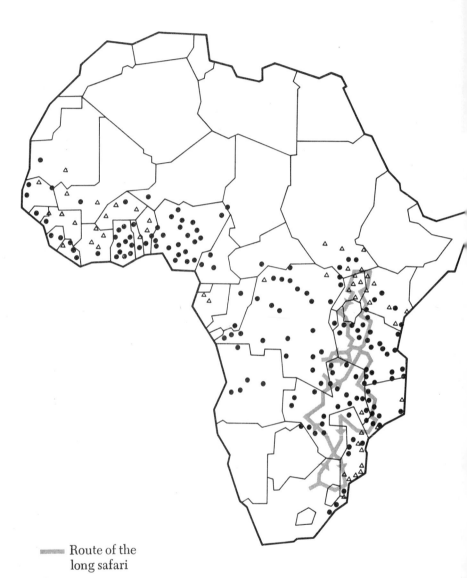

▬ Route of the
long safari

● Areas where there are several cases.

△ Areas where the tumour is known to be common but where there is no
specific documentation.

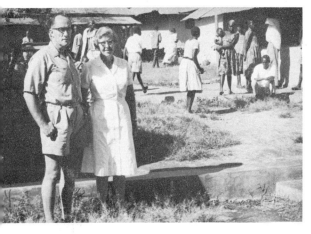

Dr. and Mrs. E. H. Williams in a busy section of Kuluva Hospital. In the background are medical assistants, patients, and relatives of patients who help with the nursing.

Dr. E. H. Williams (right), standing beside his Land Rover, looks across at Mount Wati in the West Nile District of Uganda. A remarkable cluster of twelve cases of Burkitt's lymphoma occurred here in 1966-67.

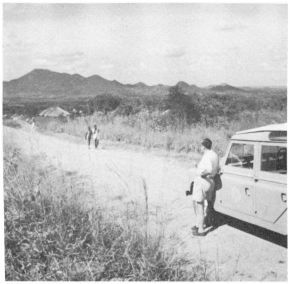

A group of twelve children (below), treated by Denis Burkitt, in total remission from Burkitt's lymphoma after chemotherapy.

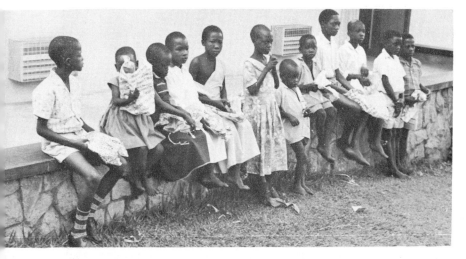

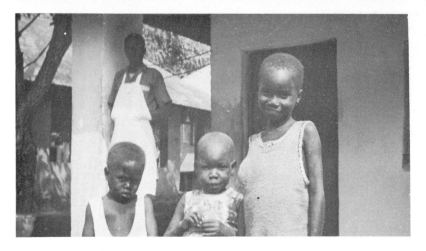

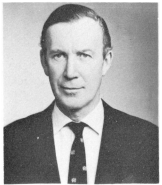

Three children at Kuluva Hospital who responded extremely well to a new method of treatment discovered by Dr. E. H. Williams, combining cytoxan (cyclophosphamide) with potassium iodide. The taller boy, on the right, was a very severe case: He had a jaw tumor, a spinal tumor which caused complete paralysis, a tumor in a leg bone, and later a tumor of the orbit of the eye. At the time the photograph was taken he had been in complete remission for twelve months.

Mr. Peter Clifford

Mr. Peter Clifford, of Kenyatta National Hospital, Nairobi, with a group of fifteen children, all of whom are in "total tumor regression" from Burkitt's lymphoma as the result of treatment by chemotherapy and, in some cases, immunotherapy. Some of the children still show signs of bony deformities, which can be expected to improve with time.

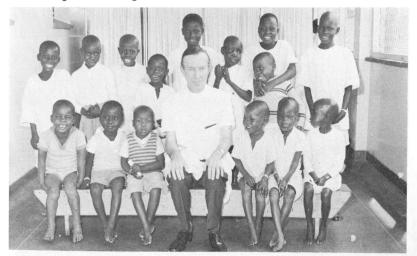

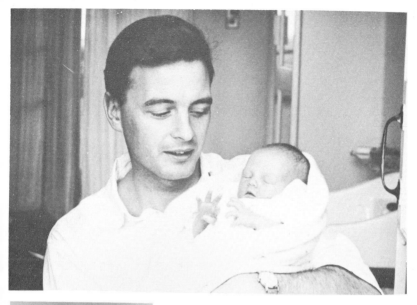

Dr. Dennis H. Wright
with his sixth child, Margaret,
who was born in Kampala in 1964.

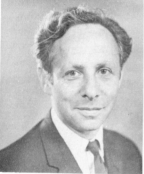

Professor M. A. Epstein

A group of "immature"
EB virus particles in an infected
cell. The magnification of this
electron micrograph is 119,000.

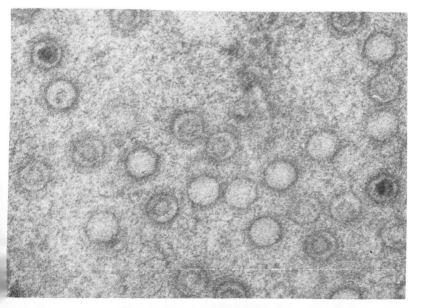

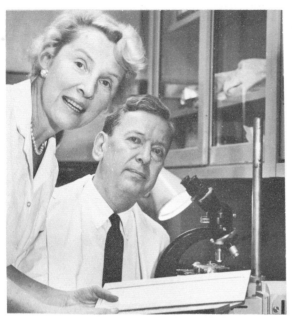

Drs. Gertrude and Werner Henle.

Dr. Werner Henle addressing the technical assistants who worked on the Burkitt-infectious mononucleosis project. They are, from left to right, Evelyn Walters, Elaine Hutkin, Theresa Berry, Angelika Patzel, and Marie Adams. Dr. Gertrude Henle stands listening in the background.

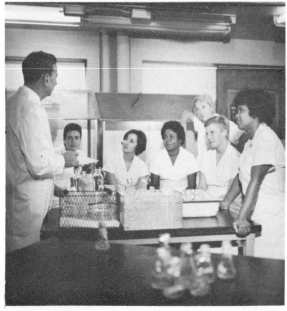

11

The African *Lymphoma?*

The air is clear in Kampala, the temperature is moderate, the streets are broad, the government buildings are dignified, and some of the better residential areas remind the American visitor of sections of Washington—the houses are set in spacious grounds, with delightful gardens. An English visitor might be reminded, perhaps, of one of his cathedral towns, Exeter, or Salisbury. In general, the city is placid. Nothing very much happens. Every evening the young Asians turn out in all their finery to parade along the main thoroughfare, Kampala Road; and every evening, also, precisely at sundown, an immense population of fruit bats flutters over the city to raid the orchards on Lake Victoria. The huge creatures fill the sky. There are millions of them. Then, at daybreak, they fly back to their roosts in Bat Valley, near the university.

One cannot claim that the city's quietude was greatly disturbed by Mr. Burkitt's bombshell. Few of its citizens were aware that anything noteworthy had occurred at Mulago Hospital or Makerere University College Medical School.

E

Insiders, however, were well aware of it. There was a great upsurge in activity, a great sense of excitement. One of the scientists who was in Kampala at the time, and who has since returned to take up an appointment at a large English university, said recently, "We were really under enormous pressure out there. Makerere is a small university, but with only one quarter of the staff that I now have here in England we were doing four or five times more work. I can remember working in the lab until nine, ten, twelve o'clock at night for several nights running."

Mr. Burkitt's safaris, in fact, had opened a door on a new and mysterious landscape. The next stage was to investigate in detail precisely what was taking place out there; and a number of new personalities now began to make their appearance, starting a series of extraordinary new expeditions of discovery. Among them was a young scientist working at the University of Bristol.

In 1960, Dennis H. Wright, an Englishman, faced a prospect that has dismayed young men in many countries since World War II: he was due to be called up for military service. Four years earlier he had qualified as an M.D., and he had been given deferments in order to work on a number of research projects. He was married; he had three children—two girls and a boy, aged four, two, and one; but there seemed to be little hope that he would be given any further deferment. National Service—the British equivalent of the American draft—was then petering out. The public mood in Britain was markedly unwarlike; the pomp and the trappings and the responsibilities of Empire were fast fading away; but the army—whatever its size and whatever its spirit—still needed medical officers.

Dr. Wright's unhappiness was at least twofold. He loved

his family and had an aversion to leaving home; and, further-more, his interests were somewhat removed from the field of general medicine. His field was pathology, and he had spe-cialized in histochemistry—the microscopic study of the chemistry of tissues and cells. A histochemist in the dwindling British army would have little hope of furthering his career, and Dennis Wright gloomily foresaw that in terms of what he could do best, his army service would be a waste of time.

At this point his life was changed by a simple and unex-pected remark. "The consultant hematologist* at Bristol, Dr. Alan Raper," he recalls, "had been the chief government pathologist in Uganda. He knew that my time was running out on the particular research I was doing, and one day he came to me and said, 'Why don't you go out to Uganda as a lecturer in the medical school?' At first this seemed like a completely mad proposition—I'd never thought of anything of the sort; but he pointed out that the Medical Recruitment Board might accept it as national service, in lieu of actually serving in the army. I wrote to them, and to my surprise they agreed."

So, some time later in 1960, Dennis Wright, twenty-nine years old, set off from London Dock on the *Rhodesia Castle* with his wife and three children, and sailed a familiar route around Gibraltar, through the Mediterranean to Port Said, Suez, Aden, Mombasa, and then by train to Kampala. At the railroad station he found that the entire Department of Pa-thology had turned out to greet him, a friendly gesture that caused him some embarrassment. In those days he used an electric razor, but there was no provision for such gadgets on the train, and he met his new colleagues for the first time

---

* A hematologist is a physician specializing in blood and the blood-forming tissues.

with three days' growth of whiskers sprouting all over his face.

The family settled into a house on a new college housing estate called Katalemwa, seven miles from Kampala. Progress had not spoiled Katalemwa. It was still rural, filled with masses of birds—and nowhere are the birds more entrancing than in Uganda. At night there were masses of fireflies—and nowhere is the night air softer or more deliciously fragrant. On the weekends, the drums of the hill tribesmen kept up an endless beat, and there was always the possibility of an encounter with a cobra or a mamba. "The problem of poisonous snakes isn't as severe as it is in India or Southeast Asia," Dr. Wright says, "but we had them. And one of my first postmortems was on a man who had died of snakebite."

The university staff, by force of circumstances, made up a tightly knit group. "There was an active social life. One frequently went out to dinner, and entertained people or gave parties in return. Our own social life tended to be less active because we had a young family and we enjoyed staying at home with the children rather than going out to a lot of parties. All the same, it was very pleasant. We didn't feel in any way cut off. In England, university staff tend to follow a nine-to-five routine, whereas in Africa we had an intimate contact all the time. We were all expatriates in a minority community, and we shared common problems and ambitions."

Mulago Hospital surprised him: "It was housed in an old pavilion-style building. I hadn't expected to see flowering trees between the wards, or the women in their gaily colored *basutes*." Some time later, when the Burkitt story aroused attention in the outside world, a London newspaper printed an artist's concept of the scene. Denis Burkitt was portrayed as a tall, thin, bony Colonial wearing a pith helmet, shorts, and knee-length stockings, and to underline his scientific qualifications the artist had given him a Van Dyke beard. Mulago Hospital appeared as a little bamboo hut; and Mr. Burkitt stood outside it, under a coconut tree, gravely inspecting an African child for signs of some deadly disease. "It wasn't like that at all," Dr. Wright comments.

But in 1960 few European or American scientists would have been impressed by the Department of Pathology in Makerere University College Medical School. It consisted of Professor J. N. P. Davies, two lecturers (one of whom was Dr. G. C. O'Conor) and the new arrival, Dr. Wright. Dr. O'Conor had come out in 1958 and was preparing to return to Washington, leaving the department with a staff of three pathologists.

It would have been an error to judge the department by its size. A great deal of work was being done, including a surprising amount of research. Professor Davies, for the first time in Uganda, had described a rare form of heart disease called endomyocardial fibrosis (a condition in which the lining and the muscles of the heart are affected by the formation of fibrous tissue. The disease has a high mortality rate and occurs commonly in young Africans in their second and third decades). Davies and O'Conor, jointly, had done extensive studies of malignant tumors—particularly lymphomas—in African children; they had then gone on to do important research on the pathology of the strange tumor discovered by Denis Burkitt.

Dennis Wright had the good fortune to become a member of this tiny, energetic unit. His official commitments at the outset were twofold. He was a lecturer in pathology in the medical school; he was also a pathology consultant to Mulago Hospital, doing post-mortems, looking at tissue sections, and so on. His involvement with Mr. Burkitt occurred almost against his own will.

"I had a room opposite Greg O'Conor's," he says. "My first recollections go back to the period when he and Denis Burkitt were working on the two papers which eventually appeared in *Cancer* in 1961. Denis is apt to talk in a very fast and excitable manner, and my impression was of a rather noisy man who used to appear all the time and chatter away to Greg.

"When Greg O'Conor left, I didn't have a special interest in the lymphomas. I was all set, then, to work with Jack Davies on endomyocardial fibrosis. The proportion of rare forms of heart disease is much higher in Africa than it is, say, in England, and the World Health Organization was greatly interested in the problem. In fact, they were planning to set up a scientific center in Kampala for the study of cardiomyopathys [diseases of the muscular tissues of the heart]: Jack Davies was to be the Director and I was to be the Deputy Director. But for various reasons Jack Davies decided to leave Africa, and the World Health Organization project fell through.

"Then, gradually, I began to develop more interest in the lymphomas—or, rather, this interest was thrust upon me.

"What happened was that wherever I turned I seemed to be confronted by lymphomas. Whenever I did a post-mortem it would turn out to be a lymphoma.

"Obviously, it was pure chance. But people began to comment on it. I remember Jack Davies looking at me in a rather strange way and saying, *You attract lymphomas.*

"If one analyzed it statistically, of course, one would undoubtedly find that I just happened to run into a cluster of them at a particular time. But whatever the reason, they kept turning up and my interest in them kept growing.

"Then Jack Davies suggested that I ought to concentrate on lymphomas and do more research on them.

"Other people didn't agree. They said, *You'll just be wasting your time. It's all been done now. Greg O'Conor and Denis Burkitt have sorted it all out. What more is there to do?*"

"And that, really, is where I started."

Lymphoma (like leukemia) is a generic term for several forms of disease that share certain features. "*Malignant lymphoma* is an American term," Dr. Wright explains. "British pathologists more often call them *the reticuloses*." The most common are lymphosarcoma, reticulum cell sarcoma and Hodgkin's disease. They all tend to have what he calls "different behavior patterns," and they respond to different treatment in different ways.

"For example, Hodgkin's disease occurs throughout the world. It has similar manifestations everywhere. The diagnosis is made on an examination of sections of a lymph node. You will see a mixture of different kinds of cells, but there is one particular cell which is said to be diagnostic—it enables you to say that you are looking at Hodgkin's disease—called the Reed-Sternberg cell. If you have a lot of lymphocytes (white blood cells) and very few Reed-Sternberg cells it carries a much better prognosis (the outlook for the patient) than the other end of the spectrum where you have masses of Reed-Sternberg cells and very few lymphocytes."

Classifying a disease, placing it in its precise relationship to other similar diseases, is obviously of great importance in understanding and treating it. One can turn again to Hodgkin's disease: treated correctly at an early stage, it responds so successfully that many patients survive twenty-five years or more and often can be considered cured.

The earliest classification of Burkitt's tumor seemed to suggest, in Dr. Wright's words, "that it was just a curious manifestation of other lymphomas." Some cases were thought to resemble one kind of lymphoma; other cases appeared to resemble other lymphomas. At the outset, Dr. Wright set himself the task of deciding whether this was true; and although he could not foresee it, the outcome was to have a profound effect.

The standard procedure in identifying a lymphoma is this: the surgeon removes a lymph node from a patient, puts it in a bottle of formalin, and sends it to the pathologist.

The formalin, to some extent, shrinks the cells in the tissue.

Next, the pathologist removes the fixed* tissue from the formalin and dehydrates it in alcohol, causing more shrinkage of the cells. Finally, in order that it may be sliced conveniently for examination under the microscope, the tissue is put into molten wax which is at a very high temperature.

"It isn't surprising," Dr. Wright says, "that at the end of this procedure the cells have changed their shape. Of course, a pathologist becomes accustomed to these changes. Indeed, if you present him with tissue that hasn't been treated in this way he is likely to be confused."

Dr. Wright decided to turn to other techniques, a decision that eventually proved to be of critical importance. He attended the operating theater personally to collect tissue material; and instead of fixing the tissue in formalin, then dehydrating it in alcohol and immersing it in hot wax, he made use of a procedure called imprinting (and called by American pathologists *touch preparations*). "You take the fresh material before it is put into any fixative," Dr. Wright

---

* "Fixing" is defined as killing and hardening the tissue and cell elements so that they are preserved as closely as possible to their form in the living body. In practice, unfortunately, as Dr. Wright points out, distortion inevitably occurs.

says, "and cut it so that you have a freshly exposed surface. Then, very gently, you touch it onto a glass slide, and some of the cells will come off the cut surface and stick to the glass. You can then use whatever stain you choose: the cells will be spread out and much bigger than those seen in conventionally fixed preparations (because they haven't been shrunk and compressed) and it will be easier to see detail in them."

Dr. Wright's findings surprised everybody concerned with the tumor. Imprinting revealed that all cases of Burkitt's lymphoma were alike. They were not a mixture of different types of lymphoma. Furthermore, the malignant cells were not only similar and of a constant type: *they differed from the cells of any other form of malignant lymphoma.**

In other words, Dennis Wright showed that the tumor was unique—the medical phrase is *a separate entity.*

* Students of biology may be interested in Dr. Wright's description of Burkitt's tumor as it is seen in an imprint preparation:

"Stained as a blood film with the Romanowsky stains, one would see what is obviously a very primitive cell. It has a rounded nucleus, although this is sometimes deeply cleft; it has three or four nucleoli and a sort of granular nuclear chromatin. It has a well-defined ring of cytoplasm which is intensely basophilic and stains intensely blue with Romanowsky dyes; and in this cytoplasm one can see vacuoles which—if you use the appropriate stain—you can show are fat vacuoles. This cell differs from the cell of any other form of lymphoma."

There have been frequent allusions to Burkitt's tumor showing under the microscope a "starry sky" appearance. Dr. Wright comments: "You have the actual tumor cell—a primitive lymphoid cell. Then you have a large non-malignant cell (called a histiocyte) which is reacting to the tumor. This disperses itself through the tumor tissue and gives the so-called starry sky pattern. It's a characteristic feature, but it is not specific."

E*

- More simply still: Burkitt's tumor was now shown to be a new disease.

The layman, understandably, would be perfectly content if no new diseases were discovered in this day and age. We already have more than enough. In the medical world, however, the discovery of a new disease—a separate entity—is an event of great importance.

It is worth repeating a few dates, to show how rapidly (in a relative sense) the story of Burkitt's tumor developed.

Denis Burkitt saw his first tumor patient, the little boy named Africa, in 1957. He first presented information about the tumor, officially, in January 1958. His first published paper appeared in 1959. Dennis Wright arrived at Makerere University College Medical School in 1960. Burkitt, Ted Williams, and Cliff Nelson set off on the long tumor safari in October 1961.

Medical science usually proceeds at a measured pace; but interest in Burkitt's work was so great that in February 1962 the International Union Against Cancer* held a conference in Paris, the theme of which was *Tumors of the Reticuloendothelial System in Africa*. In Dr. Wright's phrase, "it turned out to be a bit of a mixup." Although everybody accepted Burkitt's tumor as a malignancy, there was a lack of unanimity about its exact nature. (Dr. Wright's findings had not yet been published, and in fact were not published until the following year.) After a great deal of discussion it was decided to call Burkitt's tumor just that: Burkitt's tumor,

* The International Union Against Cancer is a nongovernmental voluntary organization with member organizations in sixty-seven countries. It is also known as L'Union Internationale Contre Le Cancer, or UICC. Its headquarters are in Geneva.

since any swelling or lump can justifiably be called a tumor. For the time being this became its official name; later the term Burkitt's lymphoma came into common use.

But another result of this conference was that Dennis Wright, at the age of thirty-two, became "the lymphoma man" in Uganda. He says, "After the Paris conference all cases of the tumor were referred to me. If a child died, I did the post-mortem; I received the biopsies not only of all cases of Burkitt's, but of all types of malignant lymphomas. Moreover, I was now in contact with a great many scientists outside Africa, and many of them subsequently played an important part in my work."

He had occasional difficulties adjusting to this role. "Sometimes," he says, "sitting at a conference in some country overseas, the chairman would announce, 'And tonight it is our good fortune to have with us the distinguished scientist, Dr. Dennis Wright, who has come from Africa to talk to us about Burkitt's lymphoma.' And I would think to myself, *Well, that's a surprise. I didn't know there's another Dennis Wright working on the lymphoma in Africa. I wonder what he's like.*"

Another name for the disease—not an official name, but one frequently used—was *the African lymphoma*. The pattern had been established so vividly: a belt across equatorial Africa, extending as a sort of tail down East Africa. Until 1960 the disease appeared to be uniquely African.

The tumor was then found to occur in the Territories of Papua and New Guinea, a discovery that caused a great deal of excitement. As in tropical Africa—which this region resembles climatically—the tumor comprised more than half of all childhood tumors. A little later it was also found to occur in Brazil, again in similar conditions of temperature and rainfall.

In May 1964, Dennis Wright went home on leave with his family. "We were staying with my wife's parents in Norfolk," he says. "And I left the family there, and went to visit a number of hospitals."

All were in heavily populated areas: the Tumour Registry in Liverpool; the Christie Hospital and Holt Radium Institute in Manchester; the Children's Hospital and Radiotherapy Centre in Sheffield; and the Hospital for Sick Children in Great Ormond Street, London.

The purpose of his visit was to review all cases of malignant lymphoma (or, more precisely, *cases that had been diagnosed as lymphosarcomas*) occurring in children under fifteen years of age, going back as far as twenty years in some instances; and he followed a very precise procedure.

He obtained, first, all the histological sections of these cases—that is, the slides of the malignant tissue.

From these slides alone he selected those cases which, in his judgment, were not lymphosarcomas (as they had been diagnosed by the hospital pathologists) but instead showed the features of Burkitt's lymphoma.

Then, having committed himself in this manner, he asked to see the clinical notes detailing the history of each case, as well as any other relevant material—post-mortem records, photographs, and so on.

The results came as a shock to everyone concerned.

He found no cases of Burkitt's lymphoma in Liverpool. In Sheffield, he found one *possible* case. In Manchester, of thirty-two lymphomas, three were certainly Burkitt's, while another three were uncertain. In Great Ormond Street, of sixteen lymphomas, six were found to be Burkitt's. "They had the typical clinical features of Burkitt's lymphoma," Dr. Wright says. "It was very strange: they had sat in the records all these years quite unnoticed. I became very excited, reading the descriptions of the multiple jaw tumors, the loosened teeth, the multiple visceral deposits—*typical cases of Burkitt's tumor in English children.*"

Altogether, there were not very many: nine cases, in a very large population, over a period of about twenty years.

Dr. Wright's investigations showed, of course, that Burkitt's lymphoma could be distinguished from any other lymphoma purely on the basis of the "histological criteria alone" —that is, the distinctive features visible in the tissue and cells.

But what caused much scratching of heads was coming across Burkitt's tumor in *Manchester,* of all places, and in *London,* of all places. What about Mr. Burkitt's findings that the disease occurred in certain specific conditions in tropical Africa (or New Guinea or Brazil), where there was heavy rainfall and the temperature never fell below $60°F$? Gray old London and grimy old Manchester could hardly be less tropical. They are rainy, but not *so* rainy; and they tend to be cold most of the year.

And so the mystery deepened just a little more; and it deepened further as, in due course, cases were reported from the United States, from France, from Norway, even from Finland. Dennis Wright, traveling around the world two years later, found cases in India, in Thailand, in Singapore, in Hong Kong, in Australia. The African lymphoma obviously was not confined to Africa. True, only in New Guinea did it occur with the same frequency. Elsewhere, it was fifteen or twenty times less frequent.

But—and this was the cardinal point—*it occurred elsewhere.* Indeed, it seemed to occur virtually everywhere in the world, wherever scientists searched for it carefully enough; and there was good reason to wonder why.

12

Mr. Burkitt Tries Some Pills

It is possible to argue that Denis Burkitt was a fortunate man who happened to observe an unusual condition affecting a relatively small number of African children, who then paused long enough to ask himself some questions about this unusual condition, and thus happened to hit upon a new disease. Any one of a host of medical persons in East Africa might have spotted the tumor; and thus all it required was the knack of being observant, being inquisitive, being on the spot, plus a little good luck.

It is possible to argue next that a few physicians, surgeons, or pathologists, having become aware of this unusual condition, would have taken the step that followed: they would have gone to the trouble of printing more than a thousand leaflets describing the condition and would have sent them to virtually every government and mission hospital in

Africa, asking if anybody had seen this condition and, if so, would they please supply information about it.

It is then possible to argue, perhaps, that somebody would have taken the next obvious step: planning a scientific expedition, or safari, to investigate at first hand where, when and how this condition actually occurred, thus establishing it as the first malignant tumor in medical history that could be related to factors of altitude, temperature, and rainfall.

At this point, though, we have begun to stretch happenstance a little too far: we have really passed beyond the statistical possibilities of good luck. Dennis Wright expressed it well: "I think most of us would have sat back and thought, *There it is. It occurs in a belt across Africa. That's very interesting. Now let's wait, and in another ten years perhaps other people will write something about it.* . . . I can't think of anybody in medicine strictly comparable to Denis Burkitt. This was a firsthand, personal geographic search, on a vast scale. Most people would have thought it was too formidable a task altogether, that you should sit back and let the information come to you. But he went right out and *found* the information."

There is one other element in the Burkitt story, however, which raises it far beyond any statistical possibilities of good luck and equals in importance all the other aspects of his work as a benefit to humanity at large. That is: having discovered this tumor, having established where and how it occurred, having led the scientists of the world to the first human tumor that might well be related to a virus (or viruses, in various combinations), Mr. Burkitt proceeded to find the means *to cure* this tumor by means of pills—sometimes, in his own words, by just a handful of pills.

Since the condition he had discovered was a terribly

malignant form of childhood cancer, and since cancer is not easily cured, by pills or by any other means, Mr. Burkitt's story thus becomes unique.

We can survey, very briefly, the medical approaches to the treatment of a malignancy.

Altogether, four different methods are available. They may be used singly, or they may be combined; but in certain situations the use of a certain method may not be practicable.

The first of these methods of treatment, and the one most widely used, is surgery. If the malignancy is confined to a single site, and if the surgeon is able to remove it completely, there is good hope that the tumor may not recur.

The second method is radiotherapy. The radiotherapist focuses his rays on the tumor and, as in surgery, if the tumor is confined to a single site and can be completely destroyed there is hope that the patient may be cured. Radiotherapy is often used after surgery to destroy any small remnants of a tumor or to deal with secondary growths.

The third method is chemotherapy: treatment by means of drugs. In the lymphomas and leukemias where, from the outset, the disease is widely disseminated throughout the body, surgery cannot be used (except, in some lymphomas, to deal with localized tumors). Lymphomas such as Hodgkin's disease may be treated by radiotherapy; but in leukemia the physician has no alternative: he must make use of drugs. Unfortunately, in 1960, chemotherapy could cure only one form of cancer, choriocarcinoma, a strange tumor that occurs (rarely) during or after a pregnancy.

The fourth method of treatment is immunotherapy—making use of the patient's own immune defenses to act upon the malignancy. This seems to offer some hope for the future: in 1960 its clinical use was severely limited, and even at the present time its use is largely experimental.

Like other surgeons in East Africa, Mr. Burkitt had attempted to treat the tumor that bears his name by means of surgery. "It was useless and wrong," he said later. "Whenever we had a jaw tumor, we could find another tumor elsewhere. The jaw tumor was only one manifestation of a multiple tumor." So that removal of the jaw tumor only too often left other tumor masses in the child's body. Furthermore, the tumor grows with great rapidity: it doubles itself in forty-eight hours or less. Even heroic surgery—that is, surgery utilizing extreme measures—could not save a child's life.

The second of the methods used to treat cancer, radiotherapy, could not be employed at Mulago Hospital for the simple reason that it was not available. In 1960 no equipment for radiotherapy existed in Africa between Cairo, in the north, and Salisbury, Southern Rhodesia, more than three thousand miles to the south.* Yet, in due course, immense benefits were to arise from this lamentable situation.

Drugs had been used to treat some cases of the tumor, without any notable success. Here, again, we encounter special circumstances. Uganda is not a wealthy country. Burkitt's tumor is almost inconsequential compared to such widespread and economically damaging diseases as malaria

* The first radiotherapy unit to reach East Africa was installed at the end of 1968 in the Kenyatta National Hospital, Nairobi, a most generous gift to the people of East Africa from the people of Sweden. A large part of the credit for this gift goes to Professor George Klein, of the Karolinska Institutet, Stockholm, and his colleague, Professor J. Einhorn. One of the first patients to be treated was a boy, only ten years old, suffering from Hodgkin's disease.

and hookworm, and there was literally no money available to Burkitt and his colleagues for the purchase of experimental drugs. The situation was summed up by Professor M. A. Epstein: "In the context of the total medical background of an undeveloped territory, experimental drugs would have been a luxury, particularly since there was no indication that they would do any good."

As for immunotherapy, its potentiality lies in destroying the last few thousand malignant cells after the main bulk of the tumor has been destroyed by other means. The tumors seen in children with Burkitt's lymphoma were—in 1960 and today—totally beyond the scope of the immunologist.

Therefore, since surgery was rarely successful, since radiotherapy could not be employed because there was no equipment available (at least, in East Africa), and since nobody had achieved any success with drugs, Burkitt's tumor in 1960 was, to all intents and purposes, a wholly incurable disease.

Chemotherapy enters the Burkitt story in the way we have come to expect. Once more the sequence of events appears to depend on good fortune. There is no great Chemotherapy Program, there are no lengthy Chemotherapy Studies, not even one laboratory mouse, rat, hamster, or rabbit is involved. There is just another unexpected and almost unbelievable step forward.

What happened was that in January 1960 a number of scientists from the Sloan-Kettering Institute for Cancer Research in New York went out to Nairobi to treat various forms of cancer with new drugs and new techniques. One of the members of this group was Dr. Joseph H. Burchenal, an authority on cancer chemotherapy. The group as a whole was working at the Kenyatta National Hospital with Peter Clifford, Kenya's most eminent surgeon.

In the course of this visit Dr. Burchenal made a trip to Kampala and met Denis Burkitt at Mulago Hospital. Some time later Dr. Burchenal said in an interview, "I thought I had seen all childhood tumors in Memorial Hospital (New York) during the past twelve or fourteen years, but I had never seen anything like these tumors. Actually, it turned out later on, when I went through the records, that I had seen some cases which might be considered to be what we now call Burkitt's lymphoma, but we had not recognized them as such,"—a state of affairs in no way surprising, and reminiscent of Dennis Wright's discoveries in Manchester and London.

The outcome of the meeting was that Dr. Burchenal gave Mr. Burkitt a drug called methotrexate, and advice on how it should be administered. Subsequently another Sloan-Kettering scientist, Dr. Herbert F. Oettgen, came out to East Africa and, in Burkitt's words, "guided me a lot in those early days."

Then, undoubtedly to everybody's astonishment, the drug treatment began to show results. A brief paragraph in the Seventh Biennial Report of the Sloan-Kettering Institute, for the years 1959–61, gives what is probably the first indication that the group in East Africa had observed something unusual: "Methotrexate is being used in the treatment of round cell sarcoma of the face in African children in Nairobi and Kampala. Definite regression has been seen in some of the tumors, and it appears that the prolongation of survival time may have been achieved."

Almost from the outset it was apparent that the tumor, in Burkitt's words, was "incredibly amenable to treatment," and the official statement, *It appears that prolongation of survival time may have been achieved,* was too modest. Prolongation of survival time in the lymphomas and leukemias is usually reckoned in months; but *six years* after he began to use chemotherapy Mr. Burkitt could declare, "Some of the first patients we ever treated are still alive and well and, I believe, cured." Some of them were still alive and well *nine* years later.

The nub of the matter, the reason for all the excitement, is that before Dr. Burchenal and Mr. Burkitt met in 1960 only one form of cancer could be cured by chemotherapy: choriocarcinoma. Two scientists, Dr. Roy Hertz and Dr. Min Chiu Li, working in 1956 at the National Institutes of Health in Bethesda, Maryland, had treated a hundred and ten women suffering from choriocarcinoma with methotrexate, and thereby had made medical history: five years later, seventy of these women were still in remission from the disease and were considered to be cured.

But the treatment of choriocarcinoma is very severe. The drug must be administered in amounts that come close to causing general poisoning of the patient. This, in fact, has always been considered to be essential in the treatment of cancer by drugs: the maximum dosage the patient can tolerate has to be given to ensure that the greatest possible number of malignant cells are destroyed.

Burkitt's experience was different. He says, "The experts told me to treat my patients very heavily, with numerous courses of the drug, but several factors prevented me from doing this. I had a lot of other things to do—I had a whole surgical unit on my hands—and so I wasn't treating patients anything like as intensively as the experts recommended. Just the same, my patients did remarkably well. . . . The initial response was dramatic. If we had relatively small tumors, we saw them disappear. If they were bigger tumors they would partially disappear: we would keep treating them and they would keep recurring. . . . We didn't know our real results for some time because although we had initial success with so many of our patients, they went away and never came back to the hospital. They might still be alive—we don't know. We had no follow-up program then (that is, keeping a record of the patient's progress after treatment). We'd started something, with no idea where it was going to lead; and we just allowed the patients to go home, and lost touch with them."

Two of these children remain clearly in Burkitt's memory. They are identified as numbers in a series—J95 and J76; and this is how it is convenient for them to appear in the official records, J indicating a jaw tumor. But in real life J95 was a little boy, about five years old, named Kibakola, and he was one of the first children at Mulago Hospital to be treated with the marvelous drug brought to Africa by the eminent American cancer scientist.

"Three months after his treatment began, Kibakola was still alive *and still well,*" Burkitt says. "We thought this was colossal, because the disease usually progresses so very rapidly. Then time went on, and Kibakola *remained* well, and his condition became more and more encouraging." He is still well as this is written, nearly ten years later.

J76 was equally encouraging, and perhaps even more remarkable.

"Some of the patients who did best," Burkitt explains, "were those who ran away from the hospital during their treatment"; and this is what occurred with J76, a little girl of about the same age as Kibakola, whose name—an unusually sweet and musical name—was Namusisi.

"I thought Namusisi would be a very favorable patient to treat, that she might respond well. She was going to have three courses of methotrexate—a full course consists of forty pills, given at the rate of eight pills a day for five days. But when she'd had only one course, her mother came to the hospital during the night and took her home. This is something that happens frequently in Africa; they are frightened of hospitals and doctors. I was very disappointed. It seemed that we'd missed an opportunity to help the child.

"Then, about a year later, one of our African workers came across Namusisi in her home in the bush. I've seen her frequently since then: she's perfectly well, and I think we can say she's cured—on only one course of pills. She lives about twelve miles from Kampala, and anyone who's interested can drive out to visit her."

The manner in which an early jaw tumor responds to chemotherapy is remarkable beyond belief. No other childhood tumor responds with such speed, and for some scientists this tremendous response is diagnostic, a certain sign that the disease is indeed Burkitt's lymphoma. Dr. Ted Williams recalls that in January 1965 a conference on the lymphoma was held in Kampala. "People came from all over the world. At the beginning of the conference, Denis brought out a little boy suffering from the tumor who had received no treatment. Chemotherapy was started then and there, and at the end of the conference, five days later, Denis brought out the same little boy again. In those few days the tumor had gone right down.

"At this conference, too, Denis had gathered together all of his long-term survivors. When the delegates left the conference room for a tea break the children were outside, wandering around for the delegates to see: a bottle of Pepsi in one hand, and in the other hand photographs of themselves showing the tumor before chemotherapy was started."

Simple demonstrations of this kind have a stunning effect upon any audience of cancer scientists. Suddenly, the hopes and the dreams of half a century of intensive research are visible and tangible: the wild hope, the wild dream that cancer can be cured. And cured not by the mutilating knife, not by tissue-destroying radiation, but by a hundred pills or less, taken every four hours for less than a week. Burkitt's lymphoma, manifested in the jaws of a child, can be almost unbearably brutal: a huge out-thrusting mass, cruelly distorting the child's face, putting intense pressure upon an eye. But *caught at an early stage* there is a good possibility that the huge mass can be reduced, the frightened child can be saved.

It is only this disease, this particular lymphoma, that responds at present so dramatically. All the same, the implications are inescapable. If one form of cancer will respond like this to chemotherapy, it may be a portent of things to come. And in any audience of cancer scientists you can sense the thoughts going through their minds as Mr. Burkitt talks to them and shows them his color slides: *Burkitt's lymphoma is in some way related to other lymphomas. It is related also, in some way, to leukemia. Leukemia! If we could treat leukemia with a handful of pills, that would be something!*

Burkitt could not expect the Sloan-Kettering Institute for Cancer Research to provide him with an endless supply of drugs. Nor could Mulago Hospital supply them: like colored mapping pins, they were not included in his budget. In typical Burkitt fashion he went directly to the Nairobi representative of Lederle Laboratories, the manufacturers of methotrexate, and (in his own words): "I told Mr. Innes that we had a cancer that was responding to chemotherapy, and this would provide a good opportunity to test his drug *because we had no X-ray therapy*. Could we have samples to try out? If they worked successfully, there were good prospects of the government placing orders for the drug."

Mr. Innes and Lederle Laboratories listened sympa-

thetically, and to their everlasting credit were most coopera-
tive. "I was given the methotrexate for nothing," Mr. Burkitt
says. "I acknowledge it to them. They gave me free supplies
for years."

Later, at the midpoint in the long safari, Burkitt visited
the huge Baragwanath Nie-Blanke Hospitaal in Johannesburg—the largest hospital in the Southern Hemisphere—and
learned about another valuable drug, cyclophosphamide
(also known as Cytoxan, or Endoxan). On his return to
Kampala, the German manufacturer Asta-Werke gave him
"liberal amounts." Cyclophosphamide is descended from the
deadly war gas, nitrogen mustard, used in World War I. Its
action is different from methotrexate, but it produces the
same striking results.

Later still, the American pharmaceutical company Eli
Lilly gave him free supplies of a very expensive drug, vin-
cristine, which is derived from the periwinkle plant.

How, precisely, does a surgeon without research funds
obtain unlimited supplies of expensive drugs? Mr. Burkitt's
explanation is simple and cheerful, and should encourage
others who find themselves in a similar situation: "Oh, I
suppose I nagged at people a bit. When you're enthusiastic
about something, you can't help driving away at it."

In fact, there was something a little more persuasive in
Burkitt's approach than nagging, and it is contained in the
phrase "I told Mr. Innes . . . this would provide a good
opportunity to test his drug *because we had no X-ray
therapy.*"

The medical significance of this remark is that X-ray
therapy affects a patient's response to drugs in an unpredict-
able manner. Therefore, if a patient has received X-ray
therapy it is impossible to obtain an accurate assessment of

the precise effect of a particular drug on a particular tumor.

In Europe and America (and, of course, in other regions where the necessary equipment is available), cancer is always treated first by surgery *or X-rays*. Except in leukemia or choriocarcinoma, malignancies are never treated first by chemotherapy. Drugs are used as an adjunct to X-rays or surgery; and thus there is little opportunity to learn what a drug can really do.

What Burkitt was offering in exchange for free supplies of the drugs he needed so urgently was just this: an opportunity—"a golden opportunity," he calls it—for various companies to test their drugs on patients who had not received any radiation therapy. They had not received radiation therapy because there was no equipment available in the three thousand miles of East Africa between Cairo and Salisbury.

The situation was tragic, because patients with malignancies such as skin cancer, which is nearly always curable by radiation therapy, had to be sent away, often to a miserable death. But the situation also had another aspect, and a man with a very remarkable kind of genius happened to be on the spot and was able to exploit it. Dr. Ted Williams points out, with great insight, "Burkitt's tumor would never have been treated with chemotherapy if there had been a radiotherapy unit in East Africa, and so no one would ever have found out how effective chemotherapy is.

"In South Africa and in parts of Rhodesia they were treating the tumor with radiotherapy, and it was very ineffective.

"The breakthrough in chemotherapy had to happen in a poor country like Uganda. It could *only* happen in a country which lacked radiotherapy facilities.

"If we had radiotherapy here in Uganda, we would never

think of using chemotherapy first. Ethically, we'd feel we must first use radiotherapy. Ethically, we must do what we *know* is best, or *believe* is best for our patients. That's the basis of our patient-doctor relationship—to do the best for the patient.

"Therefore you are always hesitant to use something untried, when you have available something that is tried and proven. When you are responsible for people's lives, you know you *might* hit on something that's better than what you've been using; but you dare not try it. It might turn out to be not better but worse.

"Our circumstances were different. If radiotherapy had been available we would have had to use it. But there was none available, and we were left with chemotherapy.

"And the chemotherapy happened to work."

Mr. Burkitt's good luck? Mr. Burkitt's good fortune? After it happens again and again, one begins to wonder.

13

The Place of Cold Water

Nairobi, in January 1897, when Dr. Albert Cook and his fellow missionaries reached it on their safari from Mombasa to Kampala, consisted of a few mud and grass shacks standing on a swamp beside the Athi River. Dr. Cook and Katherine Timpson and the rest camped there that night, but they did not sleep well. A band of Masai was nearby, decked out in ostrich feathers and red capes, carrying long spears and heavy shields, and they might only too easily cause serious trouble—a year before they had attacked a safari of fifteen hundred people, killing three hundred. Throughout the night the missionaries saw fires blazing in the distance, they heard yells and shots and the beat of war drums, but in the morning they learned that many of the Masai had been slaughtered by their bitter enemies, the Wakamba, nomadic, pastoral people who obviously were not overawed by the legendary prowess of the Masai warriors. The missionaries did not linger to witness any counterattack.

The shacks by the swampy river were called Martin's Camp. With the coming of the Mombasa-Uganda railway a station was built here and the settlement became known by its Masai name, Nairobi, the place of cold water (or, as some people have it, the place of fresh water). It grew to be the capital of Kenya, and until 1961 only Europeans were permitted by law to settle in the region. It was built by the white man to serve his various purposes in East Africa; for the most part it still looks like a white man's city; and you cannot by any effort of the imagination turn it into what in fact it now is, an African city.

It is all somewhat commercial these days, with a great many new hotels that seem to have been brought over intact from Miami Beach, but as you walk the broad and sunny streets you get an occasional whiff of the past, an occasional glimpse of ghosts who in their time were strong and vigorous and very arrogant. Sit at a table outside the New Stanley, and you are inevitably reminded of Ernest Hemingway and his bold white hunters and his disagreeable heroines and their feeble husbands—they are still climbing in and out of Land Rovers, bustling in and out of the old hotel, carrying vast amounts of expensive luggage, and huge hand-chased elephant guns, and Fortnum and Mason hampers, and the red and yellow Shell Road Map of East Africa.

The great climactic confrontations between man and beast are gone forever, though. Hardly anybody is allowed to shoot Kenya's glamorous animals—they are a precious asset, and the authorities are desperately trying to preserve them. Nairobi is a trade center and a tourist center: the bold white hunters take you out to the game parks just to photograph the animals and not to encounter them on any Hemingwayesque kill-or-be-killed basis: you may not even *annoy* them. The animals are bored to death with being photographed, the lions yawn in your face; and when you yourself have become bored with their boredom you can go shopping in the best Western style. You can buy the most expensive cameras, the finest guns, gorgeous jewels, elegant clothes to wear on safari or to garden parties; and in the charming little boutiques they will murmur in madame's ear, "Signor Pucci paid us a visit yesterday afternoon. Such a nice man." Meanwhile, the poachers, despising the authorities, go on killing the game freely, in authentic African style: silently, with the spear or the club, in traps, in pits. They need the meat. They are hungry.

If you have reason to go to East Africa, not as a tourist but on Burkitt business of some kind, you might go first to Mulago Hospital in Kampala, Uganda, and then to the Kenyatta National Hospital in Nairobi, Kenya; or vice versa. The two hospitals, four hundred miles apart, are in a sense twins: both have a very deep commitment to the strange lymphoma that has aroused such widespread excitement. Mr. Burkitt, of course, was the leading figure in Kampala; his counterpart in Nairobi, also a surgeon, is Mr. Peter Clifford, who enters the narrative for two good reasons—first, as another of the remarkable human beings who give the story such a heroic quality; and second, because he brings to it something every good story should have, the element of conflict.

Kenyatta National Hospital is in process of being rebuilt. A young Swedish cancer scientist, Dr. Jan Stjernswärd,* said

* Dr. Stjernswärd is on the staff of the famous Department of Tumor Biology at the Karolinska Institutet, Stockholm. In

of the plans for the new hospital, "When it is finished it will be magnificent, the best hospital in Africa, one of the best in the world. We have nothing like it in Sweden."

The old hospital is still tremendously active, like any African hospital. In Europe or America the entrance to a hospital is usually quiet, subdued. Here there is noise, color, endless drama. A Mercedes-Benz 230 comes screaming up to the entrance, doors are flung open, two young Africans jump out and drag out a third young African in a Madison Avenue suit who is unconscious, sweating, limp as a rag doll: he seems to be dying of—what? You cannot even guess. Young girls—they can hardly be twelve years old—in gay *basutes* sit on the grass nursing their babies and giggling. Men with bandaged heads or a broken arm, a broken leg, a broken collarbone, replay for visitors the fight or the car crash that caused their disability. A beautiful Bedouin woman, swathed in black, sits on a stone step, smiling remotely: two children play near her, a lovely little girl, and a little boy, about four years old, with the swollen jaws of Burkitt's lymphoma. A brisk blond English nurse tells you, "Oh yes, the hospital is full of Burkitt's tumor. A lot of cases."

Then, if you go inside the hospital, past the patients sitting in rows in the foyer, and turn right along the corridor, and climb a flight of stairs, you will come to the Burkitt wards. They are airy; the beds are widely spaced; everything is very neat; the children—those who are not asleep—look at you with interest; a couple, with paraplegia, sit in wheelchairs on a balcony.

If it is early in the morning, Mr. Clifford may be making

1967 he was awarded an Eleanor Roosevelt International Cancer Research Fellowship (funded by the American Cancer Society) and he elected to go out to work with Mr. Clifford in Nairobi for more than a year.

his rounds; then he has a number of operations scheduled. He is a busy man, pressed for time, but he may be able to spare you a few minutes to tell you what he is doing or, better still, what he is thinking; and he takes you into his office, which is about as large as a broom closet and contains nothing much more than a battered old desk, a couple of battered old chairs, and a bookshelf.

He is a quiet, handsome, aristocratic man, the perfect image of an eminent surgeon. His voice, no matter how long he speaks, remains at the same level, rather hushed, neither rising nor falling, and always very precise. His friend, George Klein, said of him in a mysterious yet magical phrase, "He is unique: he has climbed Kilimanjaro, but he does it every day—his whole life consists of climbing Kilimanjaro. He has a profound wish, a desperate wish to do something for these children with Burkitt's lymphoma, and he's trying everything that might help them. There are few medical men who have this as their primary motivation. In his case it is really so."

Peter Clifford came to East Africa after the end of World War II. He spent two years in Tanzania before going back to London and to Newcastle, in the north of England; then, in 1954, he returned to Kenya. He is a Roman Catholic, but he did not come out to Africa with any missionary intent, nor, he says, "do I have any missionary inclinations."

It is an idea that he finds important, and he discusses it in detail: "Many of the doctors working in Africa are people who are highly motivated and who have a great interest in the performance of their duties. This relates to several things.

"First, in England—as you know—there is a growing dissatisfaction with working conditions. It is felt that the present system destroys any interest, any initiative, that the doctor has directly in his patients. If he diagnoses a condition it is then passed over to somebody else, and in the end he bears little responsibility. This feeling of *responsibility* which the doctor bears to his patient is something that every doctor values a great deal.

"Secondly, in Africa there is an enormous field for any type of work. If, for instance, you send a gynecologist to work in Kisumu (northwest of Nairobi, on Lake Victoria), he could quite easily fill the Nyanza Provincial Hospital entirely with gynecological work. There is a vast amount to be done. And the physician realizes that very often he is the only person who stands between a patient with a painful, dreadful disease, and nothing. And death.

"A third point, of course, is that most of the patients with Burkitt's lymphoma are young children. And there is always something very pathetic and sorrow-making about a child with a horrible and ugly mutilating tumor.

"The health of the people here is a growing problem. The population of Kenya alone is increasing at the rate of 6 percent annually. We now have about ten million people, and it has been estimated that at the present rate of increase we will have twenty-five million by 1981–82.

"Health is, within limits, directly related to economics; economics is related to education. So, to enable the country to train doctors, to buy doctors from the outside, to buy medicine, to find the money to build hospitals, the economic status of Kenya must be improved; and the only way this can be done is by improved education.

"It's a circle. Obviously, the first step that will enable us to break out of it must be more widespread education, and this is proceeding—within the limits proscribed by the resources available to this country. But we are short of teachers, both in primary and secondary schools; we are short of schools, both primary and secondary; and the greater part of the population of Kenya is at present completely illiterate.

"What one must remember when dealing with Africans—or, I should say, people living in the African context—is how very little hope there is in the average man's life.

"Take, for instance, a man owning a small shamba [a plot of cultivable land] in a place like Nyeri [about seventy miles north of Nairobi, not far from Mount Kenya], and imagine that he gets a disease like cancer of the esophagus, which carries a grim prognosis anywhere in the world. Where does this man go? To whom does he turn? He has very little money—if he has any at all; and the situation easily becomes totally hopeless for him. I think that the means to provide a way out, a means to provide hope that things will be better, that things can be *made* better, is what the average person in Africa requires most at the moment.

"Or, if you drive a little further, up towards Meru or Embu, you will go through the heartland of the Kikuyu country. Try to envisage what one of these smallholders feels when he is faced with a major problem in his life, something as simple (to us) as paying the school fees of his children. How can that man, completely illiterate, completely without training, find money, find employment, find the means of improving his condition so that he can make the lot of his children better?"

These are some of the problems that affect every person of sensibility working in Africa. They are at present inescapable and insoluble. Is there any hope? "Hope is something that exists in the mind," Peter Clifford says, "and I think the people have more hope now than they had a few years ago."

Soon after he arrived in Kenya, in 1955, Clifford saw his first case of the tumor. The following year he demonstrated three cases to a distinguished visitor, Professor Mackenzie of the Royal College of Surgeons.

F

The nature of the tumor, of course, had not yet been established. It was variously taken to be Ewing's sarcoma, a form of cancer that occurs in children and young adults, involving the bones but not the viscera (that is, the internal organs), or a neuroblastoma, which often seems to originate in one of the adrenal glands and spreads to internal organs and also to the skeleton.

Treatment was in part by surgery, and in part by nitrogen mustard. "It may not have been the best form of treatment or the correct form of treatment in the light of present knowledge," Clifford observes, "but it benefited the patient to some degree."

Then, in 1960, Dr. Joseph H. Burchenal came out to Nairobi with other scientists to set up new methods of treatment: an event of considerable importance. "The original members of the team," Clifford says, "were Bob (R. D.) Sullivan, then of Sloan-Kettering but later at the Leahy Clinic, and two girl technicians. Sullivan remained here for two years; then Dr. Herbert F. Oettgen came out for two years, and during this period he visited Kampala about once a month."

Dr. Sullivan used methotrexate, but (in technical terms) "it was given as an intra-arterial infusion"—that is to say, it was administered through a catheter, or tube, into the artery supplying blood to the tumor. "At the same time," Clifford explains, "the specific antidote to methotrexate was given to the rest of the body. In this way you retained a relatively high concentration of the drug in the tumor, which the child could not tolerate unless his body was protected by the citrovorum factor."*

When Dr. Oettgen arrived in Nairobi he began to use a

---

* This is a remarkable example of medical ingenuity. The citrovorum factor is a substance found in liver extracts. It is also

large variety of drugs for treating the tumor—Clifford esti-
mates as many as fifteen or sixteen. And it is here that we
encounter the element of conflict: a technical conflict, maintained on the highest professional level, that is as intriguing
as anything else in the Burkitt story.

Mr. Burkitt, of course, had used methotrexate and other
drugs with remarkable success; and as a result he developed
some striking ideas about the way drugs should be employed
in the treatment of Burkitt's lymphoma. On one occasion,
in particular, he expressed these ideas in clear and emphatic
terms.*

"The normal approach to chemotherapy is to give the patient all the drugs you can without killing him, to try to destroy all the malignant cells, but our experience in Mulago
Hospital was that the patient did better if you gave him not
too big a course of treatment. . . .

"I repeatedly gave patients one single injection, and saw
not only total clinical regression, but total radiological recovery of diseased bone (that is, regrowth of the bone, as
shown by X-ray photographs); and my policy was that when
I saw total regression of the tumor on one dose I did not give
a second dose.

"We have seen patients go along to what we believe to

---

known as folinic acid, and it is related to the vitamin folic acid.
It counteracts the action of methotrexate, which is a form of
counterfeit folic acid. The cells of certain kinds of cancer have
an excessive need for folic acid; when they take up the counterfeit folic acid they are destroyed. Thus, by administering the
methotrexate only to the tumor, and supplying the rest of the
body with the antidote, citrovorum factor, the patient is protected to a large extent from the toxic effects of the methotrexate.

* The passage that follows occurred in the course of a conversation with the author of this book in Tokyo at the end of 1966.

be total cure after one dose, but this depends on seeing them early. In my experience, if you saw an early jaw tumor you could expect to get total clinical remission which would not recur at that site in the large majority of cases, after a single dose of a cytotoxic (cell-poisoning) agent.

"The very fact that we see long-term remissions (which we believe to be cures) following what would normally be considered totally inadequate therapy means, I believe, that the drug helps to stimulate the patient's own defenses. . . . If you over-treat the patient you may knock out more tumor cells initially; but because at the same time you knock out his defense mechanisms, you lose more than you gain.

"From ordinary observation, I would suggest that the minimum dose consistent with clinical elimination of the tumor is the best dose, and to go on giving more drugs does more harm than good."

In every respect this is an extraordinary statement. We are dealing with a malignant tumor of childhood that has the ability to grow very rapidly indeed; *we are dealing with a form of cancer, the most dreaded of all diseases;* and we have here an experienced and respected surgeon claiming that when the tumor is seen early *it can be cured* with a single injection of a drug or, alternatively, with what amounts to a handful of pills.

What is more, the results obtained at Mulago Hospital in Kampala fully supported Burkitt's claim. Relying chiefly on this minimal form of treatment he was obtaining long-term remissions* in 15 to 20 percent of his patients; and he was prepared to argue that these long-term remissions were in fact cures: "I know that you are hardly allowed to claim a

---

* "Remission" means that the disease is not apparent for a substantial period.

cure for chemotherapy in cancer. You aren't allowed to say a patient is cured until he's dead*; but that doesn't suit me. I am claiming cures on this ground: that if the patient is symptom-free after a year, some—but very, very few—ever get into trouble again. And therefore, nineteen times out of twenty, the patient who is symptom-free after a year will, I think, go on living and will not die of this tumor."

A similar claim, of complete cures by means of chemotherapy alone, could be made only in the case of choriocarcinoma. Here, while the cure rate was considerably higher, it was obtained by intensive treatment. But choriocarcinoma is a peculiar tumor; it is unique; and the success achieved in its treatment cannot be applied directly to the treatment of any other malignancies.

On the other hand, Burkitt's lymphoma is related to the other lymphomas, including Hodgkin's disease, and to the leukemias; and scientists all over the world reacted with sharp interest to reports of minimal drug treatment that resulted in 15 to 20 percent long-term remissions *which could be considered cures*. Dr. Burchenal, at the Sloan-Kettering Institute for Cancer Research, commented with deep feeling, "If we could get 15 to 20 percent long-term remissions in leukemia it would be wonderful"; and in a famous paper entitled "Geographic Pathology—Burkitt's Tumor as a Stalking Horse for Leukemia," he urged intensive study of Burkitt's lymphoma in the hope that an understanding of its features might be turned to use in the treatment of all those other related diseases.

In Nairobi, however, Peter Clifford was dealing with the problem in a different manner. He, too, was treating Burkitt's

---

* An age-old medical quip.

lymphoma by means of drugs; but, unlike Mr. Burkitt, he was using *intensive* chemotherapy.

And with intensive chemotherapy Mr. Clifford was obtaining survival rates that were exactly the same as Mr. Burkitt's: 15 to 20 percent of his patients were going into long-term remissions.

Mr. Burkitt relied, wherever possible, on a single injection, or a handful of pills. Mr. Clifford carried his treatment to toxicity—the point where the patient shows clear signs of poisoning.

Yet both men achieved the same results; and to many onlookers the situation seemed to make no sense.

Mr. Clifford's attitude was this: "A great many dogmatic statements have been made about Burkitt's lymphoma as a result of generalizing but without any real proof. Every Burkitt tumor in each individual child presents as a separate problem, and the relation of each child to his tumor is a separate and individual thing.

"In one child, with a single dose of chemotherapy you will kill off a certain proportion of the malignant cells; and then regrowth will occur.

"In the next child, with the same dose you will kill off a different proportion of the malignant cells; and then regrowth will occur.

"In a very fortunate child, with the same dose you will kill off all the malignant cells.

"But in the majority of Burkitt patients you will get this pattern: they will require successive doses of chemotherapy before the tumor cell population is completely eliminated.

"If the patients are followed up and kept under observation, you may find that this regression bears no relation to what ultimately happens. For example, you may completely eliminate all systemic tumors (that is, throughout the entire body) and yet the child may die of a tumor other than the presenting (original) tumor, or as a result of extension of the disease into the central nervous system (the brain and spinal cord).

"Again, a great number of enthusiastic and generalized statements have been made about the patient's immediate response to chemotherapy. I agree that the tumor is enormously sensitive to chemotherapy; but the aim of any form of treatment is, at the end of five or ten years, to have a live child."

Physicians often do not see eye to eye about the best form of treatment for a given malady. But here the dispute seems to go somewhat beyond the limits of a simple difference of opinion. The lives of many children are deeply and directly involved in this issue; and because of the broader implications of Burkitt's lymphoma, there could be serious effects upon the understanding and future treatment of other childhood malignancies (and, for that matter, adult malignancies).

"The point I want to get across," says Clifford, "is that the chemotherapy of Burkitt's lymphoma is not easy. And although 15 to 20 percent of patients go into long-term remissions—a most encouraging figure compared with acute leukemia—one must not forget that 80 to 85 percent are still dying of the disease. For each of those individual children who make up the 15 to 20 percent, survival really represents 100 percent survival; whereas it is no encouragement to the parents of a child who dies to tell them that 15 to 20 percent survive."

Clifford was particularly alarmed because at least two children whom he had treated in 1963, and who appeared to be completely cured, had died five years later when the disease recurred.

Yet Denis Burkitt had stated that such recurrences could be expected: "If the patient is symptom-free after a year, some—but very, very few—ever get into trouble again."

So, a problem was raised. And this problem in itself raised another problem: how could anybody possibly attempt to solve the problem? For, in the case of a child suffering from a disease that might be fatal, a physician is not permitted to experiment. In the words of Dr. Ted Williams, "Ethically, we must do what we know is best, or *believe* is best for our patients." But what is considered to be best when one expert urges minimal doses of chemotherapy, and another expert—equally committed—urges maximum dosage?

The problem and its accompanying problem-within-a-problem may eventually be solved in an ancient hospital hut in Kampala, formerly the Maternity Centre of the old Mulago Hospital and now a center for the treatment of lymphomas, principally Burkitt's. A rough wooden sign at the entrance reads:

The Lymphoma Treatment Centre
Is A Joint Effort Of The Makerere
College Medical School And
The National Cancer Institute
Of The United States
Public Health Service

This sign nailed on to the wall of a hut in Uganda requires a few words of explanation.

The National Cancer Institute is one of the nine Institutes and four Divisions that make up the National Institutes of Health of the United States, and it is the Federal government's principal agency for research on the cause, diagnosis, treatment, and prevention of cancer.

In recent years so-called task forces—groups of experts—have been formed to concentrate on certain particularly urgent problems; among these have been an Acute Leukemia Task Force and a Lymphoma Task Force. Inevitably there is profound interest in Burkitt's lymphoma, and a sub–task force was established in 1966 to investigate it. One group of scientists works at the National Institutes of Health in Bethesda, Maryland; another group is based at the Lymphoma Treatment Centre in Kampala; a third group is in Accra, where American and Ghanian scientists are cooperating to study the disease.

Following the precedent set by Denis Burkitt, members of the Kampala group visited district hospitals in outlying areas where the lymphoma had previously been reported and urged medical officers to keep an eye out for new cases of the disease and to send children to the treatment center as speedily as possible. Small sums of money were left wherever necessary to pay for transportation.

As a result, in a period of eighteen months the center admitted forty-eight patients who had received no previous treatment.

The physicians in charge of the center now came face to face with the question nobody could answer: Which form of treatment was best for these children—Burkitt's minimal treatment or Clifford's intensive treatment? Dr. Richard H. Morrow (who, in the cheerful words of a colleague, Dr. John L. Ziegler, "single-handedly built this unit up from a mud hut to the gleaming clinical center it now is") expressed the dilemma in a paper published in 1967: "The major problems of which drug to give, the best total dose (of a particular drug) to give, and whether this should depend on the 'extent' of the disease, remain unsolved. It is our belief that

F*

these problems will not be resolved without strictly controlled clinical trials."

But how do you go about carrying out strictly controlled clinical trials on children suffering from a highly malignant cancer that may kill them in twelve weeks?

The answer is, by employing a procedure called randomization.

The initial steps are routine. The child receives a thorough examination, his (or her) condition is fully assessed, and so on.

The physician then proceeds with his duties. But instead of deciding upon such and such a form of treatment, so many courses of such and such a drug, he reaches into a file cabinet, takes out an envelope, opens it, and draws from it a slip of paper (as if he were conducting a lottery). It is this slip of paper that determines, *at random,* the precise treatment the child will receive. In the Lymphoma Treatment Centre the slip of paper may say *Minimal*—that is, the treatment advocated by Mr. Burkitt on the basis of his experience at Mulago Hospital; or it may say *Intensive*—the treatment advocated by Mr. Clifford on the basis of his experience at Kenyatta National Hospital. From another envelope, in the same way, the physician will then draw a slip of paper instructing him which of several drugs shall be used; and once the slips of paper have been drawn, the child's treatment goes forward. Minimal. Or intensive. This drug. Or that drug.

Randomization, at first sight, seems to be utterly inhumane, substituting blind chance for the intelligence and the experience and—above all—the concern of the physician. It seems to be a total abandonment of responsibility; and it seems, furthermore, to be seriously unethical insofar as it implies experimentation upon human beings who are suffering from a grave disease.

But the fact is (as many researchers have pointed out), nobody really knows the "best" treatment for these children. Mr. Burkitt's treatment will result in long-term survivals of 15 to 20 percent. Mr. Clifford's treatment will result in long-term survivals of 15 to 20 percent. Both, in the present state of our knowledge, are "best" treatments, and thus no experimentation is involved.

The same uncertainty affects the various drugs used in chemotherapy. Nobody has established which is the "best" drug for the treatment of Burkitt's lymphoma. All have virtues, all have disadvantages.

Randomized treatment of a large series of patients will provide the answers—it is the *only* way, according to the experts, to provide the answers. And of course, in actual practice, the physician has not really abandoned the patient. He is constantly present, constantly alert; and if the patient fails to respond to treatment the physician can instantly resume his traditional posture. Meanwhile, this failure in itself adds to the store of knowledge, so that in due course there will be sufficient information to decide exactly how the greatest number of these children can be kept alive for the longest possible time.

Randomization. An ugly, contrived word. A disturbing procedure. "We shall have the answer in about eight months," says one scientist. Another says, "Eight years."

One of the men working on the problem in a hut next door to the old Maternity Ward is Malcolm Pike, a young South African medical statistician who sports a red beard that gives him the appearance of a rebellious pirate. Dr. Pike summed up the matter in a few passionate words: "Probably there has never been such striking progress in medical history as there was in the first few years after World War II, when scientists at the Medical Research Council in England concentrated on anti-TB drugs. They found *exactly* what was the right dose, *exactly* under which conditions people would respond, and so on. And they did this by randomization. This didn't stop the scientists from investigating each patient minutely, to see why his lesion collapsed and disappeared. . . . Today, if a TB patient walks into a hospital in England we know exactly what we can do with him because we've *systematically* explored everything about the disease and its treatment. And we will soon know when a child walks into the Lymphoma Treatment Centre whether we should treat him the way Mr. Burkitt thinks he should be treated, or the way Mr. Clifford thinks he should be treated. This debate, which has been going on for a long time, will soon be settled one way or the other."

14

A Rabbit in Entebbe

In March 1961, some six months before he set out on the long safari to Johannesburg, Denis Burkitt went on leave to England. Among his other activities there he addressed two meetings in London.

One of these is best described in his own words: "I was asked to speak at the Royal College of Surgeons. It was a depressing talk in a way, as talks at the Royal College tend to be. It was given in an enormous hall which could hold hundreds—no, thousands—of people; and there was a total audience of about twelve. After all, why should anybody be interested? A lymphoma in Africa. Terribly dull."

Mr. Burkitt is a lively speaker. He stands very erect, he talks rapidly, he has much to say, he is enthusiastic and often witty. One has no way of knowing the reactions of the twelve distinguished surgeons who listened to him on this occasion; but he made a definite hit with his second address, which was given to clinical students at the huge, rambling, old Middlesex Hospital in central London. Dr. M. A. Epstein, who was then in charge of a research unit in the Bland Sutton Institute (which is attached to the hospital rather as the Sloan-Kettering Institute for Cancer Research is attached to Memorial Hospital in New York), has given an interesting account of what occurred:

"Mr. Burkitt had for many years a connection with the Medical School here at the Middlesex Hospital because he knew the Director of the Department of Surgical Studies at that time; and whenever he came on leave, every three years or so, he gave a lecture for the clinical students. He described himself as a bush surgeon, and he'd give descriptions of fantastic cases—the biggest hydrocele, the largest elephantiasis, and so on—huge conditions which were seen in Africa and weren't seen here.

"Then, in 1961, he came and gave us another talk, and an announcement was put up on our notice board. I happened to see this, and afterwards I took it down and kept it. It read:

A COMBINED MEDICAL AND SURGICAL STAFF MEETING
will be held
on Wednesday, 22nd March, 1961, at 5.15 p.m.
IN THE COURTAULD LECTURE THEATRE

Mr. D. P. Burkitt from Makerere College,
Uganda will talk on "The Commonest Children's
Cancer in Tropical Africa. A Hitherto
unrecognized Syndrome."

"I had been working on tumor viruses, and I went along to the lecture out of curiosity.

"I listened to him, and after he had been talking for ten minutes it was absolutely clear that he had something tremendously important. It had immense theoretical implications. . . . After the lecture I asked him over to tea, and he came two or three days later.

"The important thing was his idea that the geographical

distribution of the disease indicated that there might be some infectious cause. This was what caught my imagination because I had been working with tumor viruses, or viruses that cause tumors in animals, for more than ten years.

"At that time, early in 1961, there was very little interest in Burkitt's work, and if I hadn't gone to the lecture I probably wouldn't have heard about it until very much later. It was just one of those accidents."

When Burkitt came to tea at the Bland Sutton Institute, Dr. Epstein discussed ways and means of getting supplies of tumor material. ("Tony Epstein was at my lecture," Burkitt said later, "and he immediately said, *This is hot stuff*. He saw implications in it which hadn't occurred to me.")

"The essential thing was to have material constantly available in our laboratory here in London," Dr. Epstein explains. "It's all very well having six patients with the tumor in the ward at Mulago Hospital, but you can't put sophisticated tools to work in Uganda." Soon afterwards, with funds supplied by the British Empire Cancer Campaign and with valuable support from Sir Charles Dodds, Chairman of the Scientific Advisory Committee of the Campaign, Dr. Epstein went out to Kampala and set up machinery for sending tumor samples overnight by air to his laboratory in the Bland Sutton Institute. "We went out to London Airport to pick up the material no matter what time of the day or night it arrived."

So Michael Anthony Epstein, M.A., M.D., D.Sc., Ph.D., F.C.Path., joined the list of characters in this extraordinary drama.

Anthony Epstein was not alone in recognizing the potentialities of Burkitt's work, even at this early stage. Other scientists were hot on the trail.

One of these was the great American virologist Gilbert Dalldorf, who was making important contributions to virology (the study of viruses) as far back as the 1930s. In 1947 he discovered the first of the Coxsackie family of viruses, which cause a variety of diseases, from a noninfectious form of poliomyelitis to "summer grippe," as well as many ill-defined aches, pains, and intestinal upsets.

Gilbert Dalldorf and Anthony Epstein were well aware of the pot of gold that might be buried at the distant end of this rainbow. Dalldorf, an unusually eloquent writer, had expressed it long ago: "The virus theory of cancer . . . remains a theory as far as human cancer goes because no one has found convincing evidence of a causal relationship between a virus and a malignant tumor of man. Proof of such a relationship for any one of our human cancers would have a tremendous impact on cancer research." And any man or woman who found and proved that a particular virus causes a particular human cancer could be sure of scientific immortality.

It is probably enough, in order to follow the drift of the story, to note a few very elementary facts about viruses: that they are microorganisms responsible for numerous afflictions in plants, animals, and man, such as (to select a few human diseases caused by viruses) measles, chicken pox, smallpox, influenza; that *animal tumor viruses* are, as the name implies, viruses that cause tumors in animals; and, similarly, that *human cancer viruses* are viruses that are presumed to cause cancer in human beings—the qualification "presumed" is necessary because no viruses of this kind have been identified.

There is some question whether viruses can be called living organisms. The argument that supersedes all others, perhaps, is that they are capable of reproducing themselves, and therefore they must be alive. Alternatively, they can be killed in many different ways so that they are totally inactive and unable to reproduce themselves, and it is reasonable to argue that a virus has to be alive before it can be killed. The name "virus" means, simply, a poison; but a great many viruses are harmless to man, and one writer on the subject even refers to "the friendly viruses," because they seem to help mankind by attacking bacteria that may be harmful to us.

In general, viruses are considered to be the smallest of organisms on this planet, but at least one is of appreciable size and can be seen fairly well through the ordinary laboratory microscope—the cowpox virus, about 1/100,000 of an inch in size. But most viruses can be seen only by means of the electron miscroscope, and at tremendous magnification—up to 300,000 times. The sheer minuteness of some of these organisms is hard to grasp. One researcher happened to cut a section through a cell that was full of tobacco mosaic viruses*; and he found, by calculation, that the cell contained about sixty million virus particles.

Viruses come in a variety of shapes, but essentially they are all constructed of two kinds of material. They have an outer coat of protein; and an inner core of nucleic acid. Here we have a slight complication: nucleic acid has two forms, chemically very similar but functionally dissimilar. One is called deoxyribonucleic acid, or DNA; the other, ribonucleic acid, or RNA. Thus, rather conveniently, viruses divide into

---

* The tobacco mosaic virus has a place in history as the first virus to be discovered. It causes a curious mottling of tobacco leaves; and it is so stable and resistant that it can be transmitted in tobacco smoke.

two broad groups, and we have the DNA viruses, responsible for certain diseases, and the RNA viruses, which are responsible for different kinds of diseases.

As far as the rest of creation is concerned, the trouble with viruses is that they are parasites and can only grow and multiply within living cells of other organisms. Once they have entered a cell that suits them they can utilize the cell's nucleic acid to manufacture nucleic acid cores similar to their own. They also requisition the cell's proteins to manufacture protein overcoats; and so great numbers of new viruses come into existence, each with the ability to colonize neighboring cells. The sum total of all these actions—breaking into the cell, robbing the cell of its nucleic acid and protein, the destruction of the cell, the colonization of other cells, together with the efforts of the invaded organism to defend itself and exterminate the viruses—results in the specific disease. That is, the disease is not simply invasion by viruses. It is the sum total of aggression and defense. In the words of Dennis Wright: "The disease isn't just what the baddies do; it's the combination of the baddies and the goodies."

In certain circumstances (nobody knows what they are or why they should occur) a virus may refrain from aggressive multiplication; instead, it will incorporate its nucleic acid somewhere in the cell's nucleic acid. The cell is thus transformed: its nucleic acid, carrying the cell's genetic information, now also carries the genetic information of the virus. Then, after the transformed cell has undergone numerous cell divisions, the virus may reappear and resume its virulent aspect, multiplying rapidly at the cell's expense and destroying it.

But something else may happen. The transformed cell, its normal functioning disturbed by the incorporation of the virus's nucleic acid, may go out of control and begin a process of wild, unrestrained growth; and this may lead to the disease we call cancer.

We know that viruses cause various forms of cancer in animals.

We know, furthermore, that certain human viruses will cause malignant tumors when they are inoculated into certain animals.

We also know that certain animal viruses will cause human cells in a test tube to become cancerous.

We have, therefore, a great deal of evidence that clearly demonstrates the responsibility of viruses in the causation of cancer—outside the human species.

But, at the present time, we have no proof that any virus causes cancer in man. The discovery of such a virus would have, as Dr. Dalldorf stated, a tremendous impact on cancer research; and once we were certain of the relationship between a particular virus and a particular cancer we might be on the way to developing new techniques for treating the disease.

There was gold under the Burkitt rainbow, sure enough. Not a pot of gold, but gold ore that would require patient refining.

Gilbert Dalldorf reported that he found a number of viruses, "some of which have not been identified (while) those that have been identified do not seem to be related to the disease." To this extent his results could be termed negative. However, he was responsible for several brilliant observations, which affected all future thinking about the lymphoma.

First, he pointed out that childhood leukemia occurs infrequently in tropical Africa, whereas it is comparatively common in Western countries. The reverse is true of Burkitt's lymphoma: it is comparatively common in tropical Africa, rare in Western countries. But, *if one combined the incidence of both diseases in a given area,* the rates would be the same. For example, the sum of the low rate of leukemia and the high rate of Burkitt's lymphoma in tropical Africa would equal the sum of the high rate of leukemia and the low rate of Burkitt's lymphoma in North America.

In scientific terms, there appeared to be an inverse, or reciprocal, relationship between Burkitt's lymphoma and childhood leukemia. From this simple base, some scientists went on to discuss the concept that the two diseases might, in a sense, be the same disease; that this might be a disease which in tropical Africa expressed itself as Burkitt's lymphoma, while in more temperate regions it expressed itself as acute childhood leukemia. The idea was exciting because Burkitt's lymphoma responded, in one case out of five, to chemotherapy, and there might be a possibility of finding similar treatment for leukemia. Other scientists disagreed emphatically with this concept, and maintained that Burkitt's lymphoma and acute childhood leukemia are separate conditions, and are not reciprocally related. The controversy persists.

In addition, Dalldorf pointed out that in areas where Burkitt's lymphoma is common, the population is susceptible virtually from birth to heavy infection by malaria parasites. Malaria has considerable effect upon an individual's immune system, and Dr. Dalldorf suggested that malarial infection might be a factor in the causation of the tumor, and that there might be, additionally, a secondary factor such as a virus carried by the Anopheles mosquito. But this virus, if it existed, eluded him.

✵   ✵   ✵

Dr. Dalldorf's team had its headquarters in Nairobi. Another team, under the auspices of the Imperial Cancer Research Fund, was based at the East African Virus Research Institute in Entebbe.*

One of the scientists who organized this team explained: "We built a small laboratory with Dr. Thomas M. Bell in charge. His approach was different from Epstein's. Tom Bell used a sort of amplification technique. Side by side with cells containing small amounts of virus—perhaps only one virus particle—he put cells that are very sensitive to virus. The idea was that when the virus left the lymphoma cells it wouldn't have to struggle around to find another cell it could infect and in which it could multiply easily: it would find another cell close at hand. In other words, it would go out of the back door of the tumor cell and in through the front door of the sensitive cell without even crossing the street. Under these conditions, Dr. Bell was able to pick up a reovirus."

Reoviruses in the past have been associated with various mild disorders designated, in medical parlance, *respiratory* and *enteric* (relating to the intestine). But they have not been implicated in any particular disease, and virologists were apt to describe them in a rather sentimental fashion as

* This was originally the yellow fever research laboratory supported by the Rockefeller Foundation. It is now officially described (in its 1967 Report) as "one of the self-contained departments of the General Fund Services of the East African Community (recently the East African Common Services Organization). . . . Most of the Institute's expenditure is met by contributions from the Governments of Kenya, Uganda and Tanzania, with a generous matching grant from the British Government. The Government of Zanzibar also makes a valuable contribution." The Institute now has full control of all investigations into Burkitt's lymphoma in the West Nile District.

viruses without a home of their own, or orphans. From Respiratory and Enteric Orphans came the prefix *reo;* and in the course of time three distinct forms were found, known as type 1, type 2, and type 3. It was the latter, reovirus type 3, that Dr. Bell consistently found in Burkitt's tumor.

The precise relationship of reovirus type 3 to Burkitt's lymphoma remains to be established. Some authorities, such as the distinguished Australian virologist Professor N. F. Stanley, believe it plays an active part in causing the tumor. Other authorities have not found convincing evidence that the virus is active in causing Burkitt's lymphoma. But the story does not end there, in polite disagreement. Once more the story line breaks away and we are confronted by completely unexpected developments.

In the course of his experiments in Entebbe, Dr. Bell—an amiable young Scottish virologist who lectured at the University of Aberdeen before coming to Uganda—inoculated a rabbit with several large doses of reovirus type 3.

Eight months after the first inoculation the rabbit was found to have a large mass on its neck.

Dennis Wright has described the events that followed:

"Dr. Bell and his colleague Dr. G. M. R. Manube brought this rabbit over to me in Kampala; and Tom Bell said, 'Here's a rabbit with a big lump on the front of its neck.'

"Rabbits aren't as meek as they are made out to be. They often fight among themselves, and when they do so they tend to inoculate a bacterium which grows into a sort of lump. I thought Tom Bell's rabbit had a similar kind of lump—I'd seen examples of it frequently in the past.

"They left the rabbit with me and went off to talk to somebody else in the Medical School. I examined the rabbit, and to my amazement it turned out to have a lymphoma in the neck and lots of deposits elsewhere. I very quickly made an imprint for examination under the microscope, and then I went off posthaste to tell Dr. Bell and Dr. Manube that this was really most exciting and it looked as if they had hit the jackpot. We did a number of things: we prepared tissue for electron microscopy, we froze down some of the tissue; but the most important and the most immediate thing to do was to put some of the lymphoma into newborn rabbits so that the tissue could keep growing.

"There were no newborn rabbits in the Medical School. But as luck would have it, one of my children's pet rabbits had produced a litter the day before. So, at lunchtime I went home and bribed the children to let me have the newborn rabbits. I couldn't move them, of course—they were in a hutch in my garage—and I had to take all the materials and inject the rabbits at home. We were able to maintain the tumor, and after that we kept breeding rabbits, so there was no shortage."

The jackpot, as Dr. Wright called it, would have been the discovery that Dr. Bell's rabbit, after inoculation with reovirus type 3, had developed Burkitt's lymphoma or something very close to it. But this turned out not to be the case. The lump was eventually identified as a myeloma (which means a tumor arising from tissue in the bone marrow) or plasma cell tumor.

A few technicalities are unavoidable here. Briefly, plasma cells are cells, found in the blood plasma, which produce antibodies; and antibodies are a major component of the body's defenses against infection. Dr. Bell and Dr. Wright, and their colleagues, now had a tumor which could be made to produce any kind of antibody. Furthermore, study of the tumor might reveal how antibodies are made.

There was another aspect to the discovery. Antibodies are constructed of proteins. Study of the tumor might lead to an understanding of protein formation. ("One of the world's leading protein scientists," Dr. Bell said happily, "would sell his soul for one gram of this plasma cell tumor.")

The greatest significance of the discovery is this: antibodies are indispensable to the body's defenses against infection, but occasionally something goes wrong in the immune system and cells or antibodies may act *against* rather than in defense of the body. The result may be an *autoimmune* disease. With knowledge acquired from study of the plasma cell tumor (which may or may not have been caused by the reovirus type 3 found by Dr. Bell in Burkitt's lymphoma), scientists may learn how to treat or alleviate many of the autoimmune diseases that plague vast numbers of human beings, such as rheumatoid arthritis or asthma. "It could mean a major breakthrough," says Dennis Wright, a cautious man, "in protein chemistry and antibody studies." The benefits, the potentialities, are enormous.

In London, meanwhile, Anthony Epstein went a different way and whipped up some excitement of his own.

15

Man Meets EBV

The Bland Sutton Institute in London is not one of the showplaces of contemporary medical science. It does not gleam, it does not impress. It is reached (at least from one direction) by proceeding through a sort of elongated boiler room under the Middlesex Hospital; the Institute lies somewhere up and beyond—rather gray, rather dismal, putting the visitor in mind of an abandoned wing of Wuthering Heights. But what it lacks in chrome and stainless steel it makes up in certain rare and intangible qualities, notably brains, energy, and vision.

Bland Sutton, in the person of M. A. Epstein, made its acquaintance with Mr. Burkitt by sheer good fortune in March 1961. Thereafter Dr. Epstein went to Kampala and arranged for biopsy samples—that is, tissue taken from the tumor—to be sent to him by air.

His tactics were quite different from those of Dr. Bell at the East African Research Institute in sunny Entebbe. Bell had decided upon a sort of cell-amplification technique. Ep-

stein set about trying to grow the cells in tissue culture—
that is, in vessels containing the requisite nutrients, maintained at the correct temperature, and so on. Superficially
this sounds easy enough; it was in fact exceedingly difficult, because Epstein was attempting something that had not
hitherto been accomplished.*

"For two years we tried to get these things to grow," Dr.
Epstein says. "I tried twenty-four different samples, without
success. Obviously, we were doing the wrong things in all our
efforts. But eventually, if you go on hard enough, you see
your way through; and in 1963 we were able to get the first
of the biopsy samples to grow. It is still [in 1968] growing
in our laboratory: it recently passed its fourth birthday. The
child from whom the cells came is long since dead, but his
cells are going on, and in a way this is a form of immortality."

Once the technique of growing the cells in tissue culture
was established there was a widespread demand for samples
from scientists eager to investigate them. Dr. Epstein's records for a short period in 1963, for example, show shipments
to Canada, the United States, the USSR, Czechoslovakia,
Israel.†

* The technical explanation, in Dr. Epstein's words, is that
"up to this time nobody had ever grown members of the human
lymphocytic series of cells in continuous tissue culture, and
Burkitt's tumor is composed of malignant cells of this type."
Lymphocytes can be described as white blood cells formed in
the lymph nodes, the spleen, and other lymphoid tissue throughout the body.

† The nonscientific reader, who may be disturbed by the
thought of cancerous cells traveling all over the world, is hereby
assured that no health hazard is involved. Persuading the cells
to grow in the laboratory, as Dr. Epstein explained, requires
special technology, as well as loving tender care; outside laboratory conditions the cells die only too quickly. On flights from

Grants from the National Cancer Institute, in 1963, enabled Dr. Epstein to expand his laboratory; Dr. Yvonne Barr joined him, to work on the lymphoma; and as a result of this conjunction the first line of Burkitt tumor cells grown at the Bland Sutton Institute was given the code designation EB_1 (*E* standing for Epstein, *B* for Barr). "It was simply a piece of laboratory shorthand," Epstein explains. "We used it for purposes of identification—for labeling our bottles, among other things." Future cell lines were designated EB_2, and so on, up to EB_7.

The Bland Sutton researchers could now go to work on electron microscope studies, and very soon it became apparent that the Burkitt cells were carrying a virus. "We were able to identify the *kind* of virus," Dr. Epstein says, "but not exactly what it was. That is, we knew the family: it was one of the herpes group. But it wasn't any *known member* of the herpes group."

The herpes group of viruses resemble each other somewhat in form, but they vary considerably in their effects, particularly on human beings. The name is derived from the Greek *herpein,* to creep (thus, *herpeton,* a snake); and the herpes viruses tend to manifest themselves in creeping eruptions in one form or another. Pigs, horses, cattle, monkeys, all have their own specific herpes viruses; until recently there were only three that were known to affect man. The most familiar

---

one country to another the cells are in liquid suspension, within a metal canister; they travel in the cabin with the crew, since if they were put in the luggage compartment they would freeze and die.

In the laboratory one sees flasks partially filled with slightly brownish broth, usually rather cloudy. The cloudiness is caused by Burkitt tumor cells clinging together in clumps.

is the kind that causes chickenpox—the varicella virus; but the same virus may behave in a different way—it is then called herpes zoster—and cause shingles, an infection characterized by small eruptions that follow the course of a nerve, resulting in severe and persistent neuralgia. Herpes simplex is also well known in civilized circles: it causes "cold sores," which appear and disappear for no clear reason. The third group affecting man consists of the cytomegaloviruses, which simply means viruses that cause enlargement of cells in various organs; their chief interest seems to be the salivary glands.

But the herpes virus found in the Epstein-Barr cell lines of Burkitt's tumor did not belong to any of these three groups. Epstein termed it "a highly unusual virus which had not hitherto been discovered." It soon became known as the Epstein-Barr virus; and this, very quickly, was abbreviated to EBV.

EBV was a remarkable discovery. Yet anybody talking about it, or writing about it, had to exercise considerable restraint, because although it was invariably *found* in Burkitt's tumor there was no positive evidence that it *caused* Burkitt's tumor. It was interesting. It was exciting. But one could not point to it (or, for that matter, to any other virus) as the cause of any form of human cancer. "No herpes virus," Dr. Epstein says, "has ever been implicated in any kind of malignant disease. And, besides, they are DNA viruses, whereas the viruses that cause all the known malignancies in animals, such as the lymphomas and leukemias of mice and chickens and cats are RNA viruses."

A technicality of some importance.

Any reader who thinks he is going to be bored to death by a dissertation on viruses is advised to hang on to his seat.

Something quite startling and unexpected is on the way. *Nobody* expected it. It came clear out of the blue.

The story now crosses the Atlantic, to the Virus Laboratories of the Children's Hospital of Philadelphia, the base of two of the world's most distinguished virologists, Dr. Gertrude Henle and Dr. Werner Henle.

"My husband," says Gertrude Henle, "is one-quarter Jewish—he had a Jewish grandfather—and he could not get a post when he finished his training in Heidelberg because of the Nazis. So in 1933 he came to the United States, and in 1937 I followed him." She is a woman who is blessed with both physical beauty and intellectual brilliance. Werner Henle is handsome, genial, and equally brilliant. They are an extraordinary team.

Werner Henle's Jewish grandfather happened to be the anatomist Jacob Henle, who lived from 1809 to 1885 and whose name was given to numerous anatomical features which he discovered, or first described: Henle's loop, Henle's fissures, Henle's glands, Henle's membrane, and a dozen more.*

Finding work in the United States was no problem for the grandson of this medical genius; and Werner and Gertrude

* Fielding H. Garrison in his *History of Medicine* calls Jacob Henle "one of the greatest anatomists of all time . . . his histological discoveries take rank with the anatomical discoveries of Vesalius. . . . As a lecturer, Henle was vivid and inspiring, winning love and admiration by his sincerity and charm. He was not only a skillful artist, but something of a poet, and an accomplished musician, beginning with the violin and eventually learning to play both viola and violoncello." He was a friend of Felix Mendelssohn, says Garrison, and had a very romantic first marriage. One could hardly ask for a more admirable grandfather.

Henle were soon investigating the possibility of population control by means of immunization against spermatozoa (an idea which has recently been revived); they went on to study influenza viruses, and then did extremely valuable work on a phenomenon called viral interference (in which one virus in a cell "interferes" with another invading virus). The course of their joint career was changed in 1956 by a telephone call from the National Institutes of Health, which set them off on a lengthy program of research into cancer viruses; and this was brought into focus by Dr. Everett C. Koop (whom they describe as "our surgeon"), who came to them after a visit to East Africa and said, "Henles: if you want to work on a human tumor that is likely to be virus-induced, Burkitt's tumor is it." The world of science, as we have seen and as we shall continue to see, proceeds in a curiously non-scientific way: great events spring only too often from a chance remark, some utterly unlikely event, a wild coincidence.

The following year, the Henles received a letter from Anthony Epstein asking if he could send them the EB cell line—he had then reached EB$_2$—for isolation and identification of any virus it carried. The Henles agreed, but their first efforts were unsuccessful. They were unable to isolate a virus by any of the conventional methods.

Now, any "foreign" organism that succeeds in invading the body is met, as a rule, by special particles designed to attack and destroy that particular invader. These particles, of course, are the antibodies, and it has been estimated that an adult human carries some ten thousand different kinds. The important fact, in this context, is that each kind of antibody is specifically tailored to attack a specific invader: if some organism invades the body, and no antibody exists to challenge it, the appropriate antibody is quickly manufactured.* We start our lives with so-called maternal antibodies, acquired from our mother; these serve to protect us for our first six months or so, and gradually disappear. Then, as we encounter our various micro-enemies we form an ever-growing collection of antibodies to deal with them. From this it follows that the presence of a certain antibody in our blood serum implies that at some time or another we have had an encounter with the foreign organism which that antibody was designed to combat.

The Henles, after their initial failure to isolate a virus from the EB$_2$ cells, argued that if there *was* a virus, and if this virus had anything to do with Burkitt's lymphoma, then a patient with the lymphoma should possess antibodies to the virus.

This very far-reaching assumption proved to be correct. Using a technique called immunofluorescence, in which antibodies receive a coating of a fluorescent dye and can thus be seen by ultraviolet rays in a special microscope, the Henles were able to select individual cells that had attracted fluorescent antibodies, and these cells were found to be "loaded" —as Werner Henle says—with viruses.

Like Dr. Epstein, the Henles were unable to make a precise identification. Almost certainly they were herpes viruses, but they did not match any known *human* herpes virus, nor did they match any known *animal* herpes virus. The safest thing to say about them was they were *herpes-like* viruses.

Investigations now showed that this virus was found, without fail, in every Burkitt patient. *Every child with Burkitt's lymphoma had the Epstein-Barr virus.*

This was a hopeful and encouraging sign. EBV, one

* Microorganisms and chemical substances that provoke the manufacture of a specific antibody are called antigens.

could say with confidence, seemed to be *associated* with Burkitt's lymphoma.

But now came the first shock.

The Henles continued to find antibodies to EB virus.

They found the antibodies, in fact, almost anywhere they looked.

And the people carrying these antibodies were generally perfectly healthy normal human beings.

Up to 85 percent of all people tested, Africans, Americans, and Europeans, had EBV antibodies, showing without any possibility of a doubt that at some time in their lives they had been infected by the Epstein-Barr virus; and no matter how far you went from civilization, the virus was still prevalent.

Men and women living on lonely farms in Iceland had antibodies to the EB virus.

The Tirio Indians, deep in the forests of Brazil, four hundred miles north of the Amazon, had antibodies to EB virus.

And about the only thing you could say about it with any measure of confidence was that it was primarily a human virus. It was not found in animals. But even this generalization was not altogether true because there is an infectious disease of chickens called Marek's disease, which seems to be caused by a virus that is, in Dr. Epstein's words, "indistinguishable from the agent we have here in Burkitt's tumor." *
Not EBV, perhaps, but very, very similar.

Virologists call a virus which has a very broad distribution *ubiquitous.* The Henles believed that a virus found so fre-

---

* This disease was first described by a scientist named Marek about sixty years ago. It involves lymphomas of the nerve trunks and various organs; it is highly infectious, and a serious economic hazard for poultry farmers.

quently in human beings must be responsible for some human disease and, in their own words, "We started to look for a disease to fit the virus." Burkitt's lymphoma was still present in their minds, but the principal locale of Burkitt's lymphoma is tropical Africa, although rare cases occur elsewhere. The Henles had a ubiquitous virus, and they were looking for a ubiquitous disease.

It was waiting for them on their own doorstep.

Working in their laboratories in Philadelphia was a technician named Elaine Hutkin. At the time of these events she was nineteen years old—an exceptionally pretty girl, with dark hair and the neat, graceful appearance of a ballerina.

In the course of normal laboratory routine her serum had been tested by the Henles, and by a stroke of luck she had proven to be EBV negative—that is, she possessed no antibodies to EBV. She belonged to the minority of Americans who had escaped infection by the Epstein-Barr virus; and because of this she had contributed blood—in minute amounts—several times for cultures to be used in the Henles' experimental work.

Then, one day, she felt too sick to go to work. "I had chills, a sore throat, swollen glands in my neck," she says. "I felt awful—I was tired all the time." She remained at home for six days. "Then I went back to work, and after a couple of days—I was still feeling awful—I developed a rash."

"She developed a rash under our very eyes," says Werner Henle with justifiable enthusiasm. "We didn't know what it was, but she was obviously not cured. So we said to her, *Let us set up another leucocyte (white cell) culture, and maybe we will find your virus.* We took some plasma from her for another EBV antibody test; and to our surprise it was positive."

G

The sequence, therefore, was this:

Before falling sick Elaine lacked EBV antibodies, an indication that (in all probability) she had never been infected by the Epstein-Barr herpes-like virus.

She then fell sick, with distressing but vague symptoms: chills, sore throat, excessive fatigue, and so on.

After a total of eight days of this illness she developed a rash.

Tests now showed a high level of EBV antibodies in her serum, which meant that since her last test she had been infected by EB virus.

Examination of a leucocyte culture confirmed the presence of EB virus.

The next stage was totally unexpected: after developing the rash, Elaine was seen by her physician. He diagnosed her illness. It was infectious mononucleosis.

Infectious mononucleosis!

And although the evidence was derived only from this one case, it was possible to suggest that Elaine's infectious mononucleosis was caused by Epstein-Barr virus.

The Henles must have felt as if a bomb had exploded overhead. EBV was unquestionably associated with Burkitt's lymphoma—it was found in every patient with the disease. But nobody in his wildest dreams would have thought of associating it with infectious mononucleosis, which is non-malignant.

But here, at last, was a ubiquitous disease, and the Henles had been looking for a ubiquitous disease to match the ubiquitous EBV. Their problem now was to confirm and prove the relationship.

"We sat down and asked ourselves, who in the United States is interested in infectious mononucleosis," Dr. Gertrude Henle recalls.

"And then we remembered: the Yale boys."

Infectious mononucleosis, or glandular fever, was first described by the Russian, N. F. Filatow, in 1886. It has yet another name: because it is highly infectious, and often occurs among young people in schools and colleges, it is sometimes called kissing disease.

It is known all over the world. Typically, it causes the symptoms described by Elaine Hutkin: sore throat, chills, headache, fatigue. Glands are inflamed, and there may be enlargement of the spleen or liver. Unusual, or abnormal, white cells appear in the blood: these cells give the disease its name. In general, it is a fairly mild illness; in rare cases there may be serious complications.

The disease resembles infectious hepatitis (according to one medical handbook, "it is sometimes virtually impossible to distinguish between the two"). It also resembles leukemia, lymphosarcoma, and Hodgkin's disease, although—as far as anybody knows at present—it is not related to these malignancies.

Until Elaine Hutkin developed a rash in the Virus Laboratories of the Children's Hospital in Philadelphia, the etiologic agent of infectious mononucleosis—that is, the organism causing the disease—was completely unknown.

So Elaine enters medical history and joins such immortals as the milkmaid Sarah Nelmes, who provided Edward Jenner with material for the first inoculation against smallpox, and nine-year-old Joseph Meister, who led Pasteur to the treatment for rabies.

The Yale boys came to the Henles' mind for an excellent reason. All freshmen entering Yale University, over a period of six years from 1958 on, were requested to supply samples of blood, together with their medical history, for a study of infectious mononucleosis begun by Dr. James C. Niederman. Records were kept most carefully, and selected serum samples were frozen for future reference.

Through the kindness of Dr. Niederman and Dr. Robert W. McCollum, of the Yale University School of Medicine, the Henles were able to draw upon this goldmine. Coded samples of the frozen serum were sent to the Henles; and in a crucial test they were able to identify—without a single failure—all samples taken from students who at one time or another had suffered from infectious mononucleosis.

In every case, antibodies to the Epstein-Barr virus were present in the serum.

Students who lacked these antibodies had never been ill with infectious mononucleosis.

To the satisfaction of most scientists (but not all, which is a perfectly normal state of affairs in medicine) the cause of infectious mononucleosis, or glandular fever, or kissing disease, was shown to be the Epstein-Barr virus, EBV, originally isolated from cell lines of Burkitt's lymphoma.

Where did Burkitt's lymphoma stand now?

16

Twenty Thousand
Little Elaines

The Papuans of New Guinea are among the forgotten peoples of the earth. They have been isolated for centuries, civilization has passed them by, and we know little about them except that some of them still on occasion indulge in headhunting. The Tirio Indians are equally remote: they tend to hide away in their Amazonian rain forests, shunning their fellow man. The people of Uganda are more accessible; and yet, until recently, most of them spent their entire lives in the villages where they were born.

So we are surprised when we find that all these diverse human beings, as well as most Americans and Europeans, share the same lowly virus. And, as far as we can tell, *exactly* the same lowly virus: for the EBV antibodies of a Yale freshman will react to the EB virus in a cell line grown from a Ugandan child, and EB viruses from a Papuan will excite the EBV antibodies of a Londoner. One cannot help marveling at the sheer persistence of living things. How did these microscopic organisms *become* so ubiquitous? How did they reach the forest of Papua and Brazil, and the jungles of tropical Africa, and the Ivy League campuses? Apparently they are mighty travelers. They sweep in multitudes around the world. And they provoke many questions.

From the good, careful research of Gertrude and Werner Henle it is clear that vast numbers of Africans, Europeans, and Americans carry EBV antibodies, showing that at one time or another they have been infected by the EB virus. Moreover, it appears almost certain that the EB virus is the cause of infectious mononucleosis.

Why, then, do so few people, relatively, come down with infectious mononucleosis?

If EB virus is associated with Burkitt's lymphoma, why do so few children, relatively, come down with Burkitt's lymphoma?

And is there any relationship between infectious mono-nucleosis and Burkitt's lymphoma and, for that matter, any other disease?

The answer to the first question is fairly simple. Few people, relatively, come down with infectious mononucleosis, even in an epidemic, because most of us have already had the disease in some form.

We know that when young adults contract the disease, the effects range from headaches, nausea, swollen glands, and so on, to a severe and possibly dangerous illness affecting the liver, the spleen, the lungs, and even the heart and the brain.

In early childhood, though, infection with the EB virus rarely reaches the status of a disease: it is more often a vague chill, a cold, an upset stomach—nothing serious enough to warrant a visit to the doctor. These are the years when we suffer from a variety of infections; some may be bacterial, some may be described by the physician as "an unidentified viral infection." On the whole these episodes are not dangerous, and they provide us with antibodies that we can draw upon as long as we live. A familiar example is polio: most people encounter and acquire polio viruses very early in life, and as a consequence they are endowed with antibodies which provide valuable protection against poliomyelitis. They also *keep* some of these viruses, so that they continue to manufacture a steady supply of polio antibodies. But some people, particularly those who have lived in well-kept, sanitary homes, do not acquire any stray polio viruses, do not manufacture polio antibodies, and therefore require inoculations of polio vaccine (which contains polio viruses and thus stimulates the body into producing polio antibodies).

In all likelihood, then, about 85 percent of the populations of America, Africa, and Europe have experienced some mild childhood form of infectious mononucleosis, after acquiring EB virus. These people possess EBV antibodies, and are fairly secure from disease caused by this virus.

The remaining 15 percent—those people, like Elaine Hutkin, without EBV antibodies—are the future victims of infectious mononucleosis, and they may come down with the disease at any time up to the age of thirty-five or forty. When we arrive at early middle age, virtually all of us are immune.

Immune, at least, to this specific disease, infectious mononucleosis. But we have no positive knowledge that after we have reached the age of forty, Epstein-Barr virus ceases to affect us. We have absolutely no idea what happens to it, whether it ignores us, whether it becomes harmless, or whether it is capable of providing us with other surprises.

* * *

The story is very different when we turn from infectious mononucleosis to Burkitt's lymphoma.

The most significant difference is that infectious mononucleosis is a self-limiting disease. As a rule it manifests itself for a fairly short period of time—about three weeks—and then, no matter how we treat it, it gradually disappears. On the other hand, Burkitt's lymphoma is a highly malignant disease: it is a fast-growing cancer, and without suitable treatment the patient's death is virtually certain within a few months.

Some scientists have argued that EB virus may be benign in some circumstances, malignant in other circumstances. Perhaps if we acquire the virus in an unusual manner—say, directly into the bloodstream—it might behave in an uncharacteristic way and initiate changes leading to a malignant growth.

But we have another fact to consider: the striking ubiquity of EB virus. It is found everywhere. Some 85 percent of the human race has encountered it.

Yet even in tropical Africa, Burkitt's lymphoma is by no means common. Outside tropical Africa, except for New Guinea, it is exceedingly rare.

So we have here a statistical discrepancy. With such vast numbers of children exposed to EB virus, we would expect to see many more cases of the lymphoma. *If, that is, EB virus alone caused the disease.*

However, we might come within the bounds of statistical possibility if we assume that the disease might be caused by the EB virus plus *something else.*

This *something else* (Gilbert Dalldorf suggested it years ago) could be malaria. Malaria comes under suspicion in the first place because it is widely prevalent and occurs in a very severe form (it is called holo-endemic) wherever Burkitt's lymphoma is common; and secondly, because it has many strange effects on the body, particularly upon the immune system. Thus, a child whose immune system has been altered by malaria might be infected by EB virus—perhaps by an unusual route—and in this way become susceptible to the tumor.

But this does not completely solve the difficulty, for there are many areas in the world where malaria is common, where the EB virus is common, yet Burkitt's lymphoma is uncommon.

We have to take an additional step, therefore, and postulate that Burkitt's lymphoma may be caused by EB virus, plus the effects of severe malaria, *plus something else.* And the virus discovered in the tumor by Dr. Tom Bell, reovirus type 3, might well be the third factor, boosting or completing the tumor-inducing effect of EB virus.

So, to account for Burkitt's lymphoma, a disease which occurs comparatively infrequently even in tropical Africa, we can envisage a complex (and wholly theoretical) series of events which would occur just as infrequently. The EB virus must, in some unusual manner, enter the bloodstream of a child whose immune defenses have been affected by malaria. The EB virus must then encounter another infective agent, possibly a reovirus type 3. The two viruses, complementing each other, might then work together to initiate the changes in the child's lymphoid tissues that would result in the growth of the tumor.*

* In much the same wholly theoretical way we can account for the cases of Burkitt's lymphoma that occasionally occur in England and the United States and other nontropical areas. Again, we can visualize Epstein-Barr virus and reovirus type 3 as the principal infective agents. They are both, after all, ubiquitous; they are found everywhere. But the child's immune

G*

Normally we acquire EB virus, as scientists say, by the oral route: through the mouth. How could the Epstein-Barr virus take an unusual route directly into the bloodstream?

The answer is simple and reasonable, and it carries us right back to the beginning of the story, to Denis Burkitt and Ted Williams and Cliff Nelson setting off in their old station-wagon on a ten thousand mile safari to learn more about this mysterious tumor: the virus might enter the bloodstream as the result of the child being bitten by some arthropod.

Being bitten—for example—by a mosquito.

At the end of 1968 some forty scientists came together in one of Nairobi's less glamorous hotels for a roundtable confer-ence on Burkitt's lymphoma. Mr. Burkitt was there, after an exhausting safari through the Congo; Mr. Clifford was there; Dr. Gertrude Henle and Dr. Werner Henle were there; so were Professor George Klein—one of the world's greatest immunologists—and Dr. Gilbert Dalldorf, and many other scientists who have appeared in this narrative: Dr. Thomas M. Bell and Dr. Malcolm Pike and Dr. Jan Stjernswärd; Dr. R. H. Morrow and Dr. John Ziegler, as well as Dr. B. de Thé of the International Agency for Research on Cancer, which functions under the umbrella of the World Health Organiza-tion. Most important, about thirty African medical scientists were present. They encounter the lymphoma more frequently than anyone else.

---

system may have been altered not by malaria (which is now fairly uncommon in Western nations) but by some other ailment, or even by a genetic defect. The chances of this happening in temperate climates are exceedingly small, compared with those areas where malaria affects the entire population; consequently the lymphoma *may* occur outside tropical Africa or New Guinea, but its incidence will be very, very low.

For several days these distinguished scientists discussed the possibility of setting up a unique experiment.

What, in a sense, they wanted to do was to recapitulate the Henles' experience with Elaine Hutkin, but on a vast scale. They wanted to enlist twenty thousand East African children in this experiment; all considerably younger than Elaine because the scientist's primary interest was not infectious mononucleosis but Burkitt's lymphoma, which reaches its peak at the age of seven.

The plan of the experiment, as it emerged from the conference, was to set up a scheme whereby the twenty thousand children would be kept under close medical supervision for several years. The immediate benefits would be great. As one scientist said, these would undoubtedly be the best-treated and healthiest children in the whole of Africa, and an immense amount of information would be acquired about anemia, malaria, and other problems of concern to the East African health authorities.

Once a year the scientists would take blood samples from each child. These samples would be coded, frozen, and stored.

No child would be exposed to danger of any kind. On the contrary, they would be safeguarded in every possible way. But since they live in the region of tropical Africa where Burkitt's lymphoma occurs most frequently, a few inevitably would come down with the disease. On the basis of statistics, perhaps ten of the twenty thousand would develop Burkitt's lymphoma in the course of two years.

These ten children would receive, of course, the best of care. Their chances of survival would be higher than average because they would be at all times under the supervision of pediatricians and medical assistants trained to recognize the early symptoms of the disease.

However, it would then be possible for the scientists to follow the procedure of the Henles, when Elaine Hutkin became ill with infectious mononucleosis. They could compare a child's blood after developing Burkitt's lymphoma with the stored blood samples taken from the same child before the disease manifested itself.*

Unfortunately, the probability is that for many reasons the experiment will never get under way. It is too ambitious; or it is too costly; or it is politically too dangerous.

Nevertheless, sooner or later, in one way or another, the scientists will discover the precise role of Epstein-Barr virus in Burkitt's lymphoma. *Can human cancer be caused by a virus?* The answer will be a landmark in medicine, for man will then be close to cracking one of his grimmest and most baffling problems.

Then, having cracked one form of this terrible disease, he could be on his way to cracking others: lymphosarcoma, Hodgkin's disease, and the mysterious leukemias. That, ultimately, is the significance of Burkitt's lymphoma. It might lead to a whole series of discoveries, of profound importance to all mankind.

It might open the door.

* It is worth repeating the scientific argument: We know that all patients with Burkitt's lymphoma have the EB virus. If the early blood samples of a child who developed Burkitt's lymphoma carried antibodies to EB virus, then the virus (probably) played no part in causing the disease. If the early blood samples were free of antibodies to EB virus, then the EB virus was recently acquired and (probably) played a part in causing the disease. With only one patient there would be an element of doubt, but the results obtained with ten patients, or more, would provide a conclusive answer.

17

Homecoming

Burkitt's lymphoma has made an extraordinary impact upon the world community of cancer scientists, so much so that it has been said (with some truth) that for some researchers Burkitt's lymphoma has become a way of life. "I think there must be an article or a new paper about the tumor published every week," Mr. Burkitt said recently. He added, "But I can't keep up with them because for the most part they are outside my competence. Immunology, viruses— they aren't my field at all."

One cannot even begin to summarize the vast amount of work being done. Most of it, as Mr. Burkitt hinted, is highly technical; but in a survey entitled *Burkitt's Lymphoma: A Study in Medical Detection,** he drew attention to certain studies which he felt were of special interest. For example, Victor Ngu, Professor of Surgery at Ibadan University in Nigeria, has demonstrated on several occasions that a patient suffering from the tumor will show a marked (though temporary) remission when he is given *blood serum* from an-

* *Abbottempo*, Book 4, Abbott Universal Ltd., 1967.

other patient whose tumor has disappeared after treatment. The implications, Mr. Burkitt points out, are most encouraging, for if we can learn how to make use of this kind of immunological treatment, "how much more welcome would it be than more and more radical surgery."

Another exceedingly valuable piece of research was carried out by Dr. Malcolm Pike, in collaboration with Dr. E. H. Williams of Kuluva Hospital. Dr. Pike, then working in Gower Street, London ("You climb seventy-eight rickety stairs to my office at the top of the building"), was shown Dr. Williams' lymphoma maps of the West Nile district and immediately recognized, as he says, that "something very peculiar was happening there." He went out to Uganda and worked with Dr. Williams, investigating in minute detail the incidence of Burkitt's lymphoma in West Nile over a period of five years; and he was then able to show that the disease seemed to occur in a pattern of clusters in space and time— that is, there would be several cases (a cluster) occurring fairly close together in a particular area (space) at the same time. Then, the following year, there would be a sort of drift, with several cases occurring in an area some distance away.

The significance of Pike's finding is that this is the way the well-known, common infectious diseases occur. An epidemic of measles, for example, will drift from one school to another and then, perhaps, back again. Thus, space-time clustering and an epidemic-like drift supported the idea that an infectious agent of some kind might be involved in Burkitt's lymphoma. "We investigated another area around Kampala and found no evidence of the phenomenon at all," says Dr. Pike, "but it continues to happen in West Nile. You can stand on a Land Rover and see twelve homesteads where Burkitt's lymphoma happened."

Dr. Pike is a member of the Medical Research Council's Statistical Research Unit; for this work he was seconded to Makerere Medical School. He says, "Most lymphoma patients get lost, and we don't know what happens to them. We decided to look at all cases treated at Mulago Hospital in the past five years, and we employed two medical assistants to help us, Mr. Josiah Mafigiri and Mr. Aloysius Kisuule.

"Mr. Kisuule is a Muganda, of the race of Buganda, and he speaks probably every language in Uganda. We sent him out to find all the patients who hadn't reported back to the hospital—about eighty, altogether; and we knew that this was a quite impossible task, it just couldn't be done. Well, he found seventy-seven of them. We wanted, for instance, to find a boy who'd given his address as Msambya Hill, two miles outside Kampala. Aloysius couldn't find the boy there, so he simply sat down on a convenient spot, and whenever anybody passed he'd ask if they had seen a boy with a swollen jaw. After he'd sat there for a week a passer-by remembered the boy, and Aloysius tracked him down to a place called Kimuli, ninety miles away."

This, too, is cancer research. This, too, benefits humanity at large.

In June 1963, Denis Burkitt went on leave to England, and was invited to join the staff of the Medical Research Council. He accepted the offer. Then, he says, "Thanks in many ways to Dr. Horsfall [Frank L. Horsfall, Jr., M.D., Director of the Sloan-Kettering Institute for Cancer Research], I spent six weeks in the United States and Canada. We visited Sloan-Kettering in New York and the National Institutes of Health in Bethesda; we went on to Chicago, Michigan, Ontario, San Francisco, Vancouver, Saskatoon,

Winnipeg, St. Louis; and arrived back in New York the day President Kennedy was assassinated."

Soon after his return to Kampala he officially handed over his surgical duties and transferred to the Medical Research Council, a change that was accomplished without moving his chair from the Department of Surgery. From this time on his work was concerned only with geographical pathology: the role of environmental factors in Burkitt's lymphoma and, later, in other forms of disease prevalent in Africa.

At the end of 1966 he returned with his family to England. They now live in a house in Shiplake, Oxfordshire, on a road "far worse than anything we ever saw in Uganda." Coming home meant that his three daughters could complete their education; that Mrs. Burkitt at last had a place truly her own; and that in his spare moments Denis Burkitt could dabble in carpentry. And, as he commutes to his office in London, he can answer the innumerable letters he received from his multitudes of friends all over the world.

"I feel that my role in all this lymphoma business has been in a sense beating a way through the bush," he says. "In chemotherapy, now, far more efficient and competent people have taken over. They're better equipped and backed; and they will do the kind of very detailed, very thorough studies I couldn't possibly have done. The same is true in virology: I know nothing about it, and the new virus experts who are coming in will make all sorts of breakthroughs. And that's true, also, of immunology. To some extent, most of what I am likely to contribute I *have* contributed.

"Now I am particularly interested in the role of diet in disease. I go out to Africa two or three times a year. I've limited myself largely to Africa because I know the terrain better than any other; but if one is studying any disease, what happens in the rest of the world is always of interest. I had a long talk recently with the Professor of Surgery in Shiraz, Iran: I realized his patterns are much closer to ours (in Africa) than they are to Western patterns, and I would love to go out and see what he is doing there. . . . . It might be that as we did with the lymphoma we can find clues to other forms of cancer in their geographical distribution; and then we would call in the experts to test the soil, to test this, that, and the other, and work things out in detail."

As for the forces that compelled him to follow up his initial observations on the tumor, that sent him off on his safari with Ted Williams and Cliff Nelson: "I realize that unless certain things had taken place we would never have managed to get off the ground at all. I realize, too (as the text on my wall puts it), *Anything I possess is what I've been given,* and therefore I can't really take the credit for it. So many things occurred—you can call them coincidences, or divinely planned happenings, however you like to look at them—which fitted perfectly into place all along the line, that I naturally feel I have no legitimate cause for any tremendous pride in myself. In a hundred and one places the whole thing might have damped out if something exactly right hadn't come along."

If Hugh Trowell had not drawn his attention to little Africa with the swollen jaw, if George Oettlé had not said, "We don't see this tumor in South Africa," if Dr. Burchenal had not presented him with samples of methotrexate, if Dr. Epstein and Dr. Bell had not arrived to investigate viruses, if Dr. Wright had not in some mysterious way attracted lymphomas . . . the recapitulation can go on and on. Coincidences? Divinely planned happenings? Who can say?

He continues, "If somebody had described this tumor

twenty years ago I don't think it would have been noticed. But it was described just at a time when there was a revival of interest in viruses, and people were interested in Africa, and people were interested in cancer. If you put together viruses and Africa and cancer you were almost bound to attract attention.

"Twenty years ago there wouldn't have been adequate air service to get tumor material to the laboratories in England and America. We would have had great difficulty doing the geographic investigation; and so on and so on. All sorts of factors dovetailed at the right time, not only to make these studies possible but also to bring in all the people who could supply the particular and distinctive contributions that were required in the circumstances.

"But I knew nothing about all this when I first began to think about the tumor. Nobody could have suspected it."

The story of Burkitt's lymphoma is far from complete. Nobody can guess what will spring from it next, where it will lead some new group of scientists. And the same can be said of Mr. Burkitt himself: his story is still only half told, there will be more to come. "Forgive me if I reiterate two points," he wrote in a recent letter. "In any sphere of life, Fruit depends upon Root. I spring from a long line of God-fearing and praying men and women, and this I know has had a great influence on my life. . . . We have a large commentary in the house on the New Testament written well over 100 years ago by one of my Burkitt forbears. Yet I must stress, as one of my uncles said to me, 'Grace isn't hereditary,' by which he meant that each man must personally and individually face up to the claims of God on his life. What I am trying to say is that my work is in many ways but the fruit of the faith that was implanted in me. It is therefore in a sense of secondary importance. Certainly to me. . . . I may be over-stressing a point, but nothing means more to me in life than a happy home. I am blessed by being deeply in love with my wife after more than 25 years of marriage. In many respects I have been made, moulded, and fashioned by Olive. Separation, even for short periods, is far harder now than 20 years ago." And so, quite certainly, his story will go on.

One can turn, finally, to another witness; and this book will end on a personal note, with the author stepping momentarily out of the shadows in order to provide a few words of explanation. In the course of my research I visited East Africa and spoke to many of Denis Burkitt's colleagues; but I arrived in Kampala late in December when the staff of the Medical School of Makerere University College had dispersed for the Christmas holidays. Subsequently, Professor Sir Ian McAdam was kind enough to send me some of his recollections of Mr. Burkitt at Mulago Hospital; and with Professor McAdam's permission some extracts from his letter are printed here. They need no further comment.

> Perhaps if I give you a few facts, this may assist you in piecing together the jig-saw puzzle of the Burkitt story.
> After the war, Mr. Burkitt was recruited to the Uganda Medical Service and posted to an up-country station in the northern part of Uganda. He must have worked there for at least 18 months and during this time I met him at Mulago Hospital when he appeared from time to time to deliver a lecture to the British Medical Association. The subject matter of these talks was related to the disease pattern seen in his district. I recall that he talked upon spontaneous rupture of the

spleen and also on hydrocele, which was endemic in the area. These lectures were well illustrated with photographs.

In 1947 he joined me at Mulago Hospital and for the next 20 years he worked with me, living in the next door house with a family that matched my own and who today remain the greatest friends.

Mr. Burkitt by training was a General Surgeon and at first we shared not only the teaching of Undergraduate medical students but also the curative work that was carried out in the 350 beds available for surgery. It was evident at an early stage that he had unusual powers of observation and these observations were recorded by photography. A filing system was started and at our weekly Clinical/Surgical meetings he drew on his collection of photographs to show that the unusual case which was being presented had been seen on previous occasions.

This in fact was how the tumour that we know as Burkitt's lymphoma was eventually unearthed as a separate entity. These tumours had been previously reported by the Histopathologist as being neuroblastomas and I recall most vividly at a Saturday Clinical meeting his very convincing deduction that if these tumours that we were seeing were in fact neuroblastomas then the incidence of this tumour was about a thousand times as common here as anywhere else in the world. The challenge was taken up by the Pathologist and there followed a prolonged controversy between Clinicians and Histopathologists over the identification of the tumour.

The clinical observations made by Burkitt clearly identified the tumour as a new entity long before the Histopathologists reached the same conclusion. Whatever claim any authorities may have to originality in the study of this lymphoma must date after the time Burkitt had established its clinical identity.

The next part of the story follows the usual pattern after an original observation has been made. Pathologists added greatly to the existing knowledge and Burkitt in discussion with colleagues such as Professor Haddow of the Virus Research Institute suggested that the distribution of this tumour was sufficiently local to postulate an infective origin of the tumour. Burkitt, who had been making contact by letter with other workers in Africa, was now determined to go out into the field and collect information. His safaris will be well known to you and no doubt you have good photographs of the sort of area he covered. He is not one of the most practical people in the world and he does not always care for the creature comforts. I am sure that Dr. Williams and others who accompanied him on these safaris will add the light touch which is essential if Burkitt's character is to be portrayed.

... Burkitt's genius lies in his powers of observation; from a maze of apparently disconnected facts he can see the thread of relevance.

As a colleague he was the most loyal and conscientious person I have ever known. He is a practising Christian who thinks action more important than words. He left behind in Africa a store of goodwill, and I doubt whether there has ever been any doctor working in Africa who has either been better known or more loved.

Yours sincerely,

I. W. J. McAdam
Professor of Surgery

Appendix: *Three Men on a Safari*

Nearly every day on the ten thousand-mile safari to South Africa, Denis Burkitt found time to type a long letter home. It was in a sense a group letter, intended to be read by the families of all three men; and it described the progress of the expedition, the sights and the scenes and the various adventures encountered along the way. There was little mention of technical matters: scientific data was entered in separate journals. Later, when Burkitt returned to Mulago, the letters were collected and became known as the Lymphoma Safari Diary, *a document running to more than forty thousand words.*

The extracts printed here, in a very condensed form, are taken from letters which were written in the course of the first half of the safari, from Kampala to Johannesburg. It is important to stress that they were typed whenever Burkitt had a few minutes to spare—in the bare rooms of rest houses, in dismal little hotels, even by the roadside when the three men stopped for lunch. In these circumstances there was no

*opportunity to rewrite or to polish a phrase; and, indeed, part
of the interest and charm of these letters is their spontaneity.
They tell of the camaraderie that existed between the three
men, and of their deep and ever-present faith; and, perhaps
more than anything else, they reveal Denis Burkitt's remarkable powers of observation.*

Bukoba: 7 October 1961

We have been planning this trip for over a year. The prime
purpose has been the investigation of a tumour, but we are
making use of the opportunity to investigate a number of
other conditions. The Medical Research Council have provided the funds. Ted Williams procured the car from an ex-
Congo missionary. It is a large 35 hp Ford V8 American
station wagon. Just the thing for a safari like this but far too
large for normal use. As well as our clothes and personal
belongings we have camp kit with beds and collapsable
chairs and table; drinking water, spare petrol, and two extra
spare tyres and tubes. Also, chains in case of very muddy
roads, and a certain amount of food plus a primus stove.

We packed up this morning. Saying good-bye is the worst
part of any journey, but this is a sign of the love we know
follows us. We eventually got off at 9:15 on our estimated
9,000-mile safari.

Today has been a perfect day. The first 86 miles to
Masaka were on good tarmac road. The country is rather
monotonous with fairly low hills all of approximately equal
size with uniform flat tops. The grass is very long, and plan-
tains with their enormous leaves are the main feature of
vegetation. There are coffee and cotton, of course, and approaching Masaka the coffee is more profuse. The green is
broken by the bright red of the Erythrinum trees. The houses

are mostly mud and wattle; a few are of red brick with roofs of corrugated iron or red tile. Those who can afford it like to give up thatch.

The tarmac ends at Masaka. Beyond this the country becomes more open and the grass is shorter. Mango trees and euphorbia come more into the picture. Bicycles are common all over this country, but we expect there will be fewer later on. We saw many plantations of eucalyptus, planted for firewood and building poles, and passed a number of buses with the usual feature of African buses—large bicycle racks on the roof.

We had a picnic lunch some 40 miles south of Masaka. Olive had prepared a perfect meal, with everything labeled. We remarked how much better it was than a 10-course lunch at the Imperial Hotel in Kampala. We stopped miles from anywhere, and yet Ted said, "Don't let's stop in a populated area"!

We crossed the border into Tanganyika at a small place called Mutukuku. There was no road barrier, just a notice. A ferry held us up for about half an hour, but it was full of interest. A heavy wire cable crossed a fast-flowing river. The cable ran along the deck of the ferry, and the ferry was propelled across the river by a string of Africans, as it were, walking along the cable holding on to the ferry. Thus the ferry was pushed in relation to the cable. I had never seen this before. Nearly all ferries in Uganda are now motorized. A small mud and wattle building on the other side of the river was marked "Hotel Superior."

Bukoba is really very attractive, not unlike Entebbe. The little hotel at which we are staying is almost on the lake shore, with a lovely view across the lake. There are far more Arabs here than one usually sees in Uganda. We are sharing a room, with our own bathroom and electric light.

After a cup of tea we went to look for the District Medical Officer. We had been told he is an Indian. On entering his very tidy house I was confronted with the text, "Christ is the head of this house, the unseen guest at every meal, the silent listener to every conversation." I then saw several other texts on the walls. It took no time to discover that he is a keen Indian Christian and knew some of our Indian Christians in Kampala. We went through our medical questionnaire with him, and he had kindly brought the operation registers from the hospital for us to inspect. Before we left we made arrangements to meet later this evening for some Christian fellowship and he was to invite in some of his Christian friends.

Sunday, 8 October

(Sitting in the bush beside the car, about 17 miles south of Bukoba) Before breakfast we walked along the sandy shore of the lake [Lake Tanganyika]. We saw several crested cranes and returned after breakfast to photograph them.

Duties have been apportioned between us. Ted does everything about the car and is also treasurer, paying all accounts and keeping a cash book. Cliff has himself offered to be in charge of laundry.

After leaving the hotel we looked around the Bukoba hospital. Apart from Dr. Phillips, the staff seems very poor. For the benefit of any medical person reading this letter we saw heart failure treated with penicillin, and an anaemia with Dextran [a form of glucose]. This is the only Govt. hospital with doctors for a population of 600,000.

We called at an R.C.M. [Roman Catholic mission] hospital 15 miles south of Bukoba and were warmly welcomed by two German lady doctors. One was a really most experienced surgeon. I had recently operated on a Dutch sister from this hospital. The doctors gave us all the information we wanted, and insisted on showing us around the hospital and giving us lunch, although we told them that we had a picnic lunch with us. We left immediately after lunch so that we could sit under a tree and write letters. We are on our way to a Swedish mission hospital where we have been invited to stay the night.

(Later) Swedish Mission hospitals at Ndolage near Kamachumu, which is 10 miles off the Bukoba-Biharamulo road. This is at nearly 500 feet, with a lovely view. We had tea with the doctor and his wife; her sister and husband were there too. I had removed the tonsils from this lady only a few weeks ago, and she and her husband were in All Saints, Kampala, last Sunday morning when Dick Brown preached. Ted and I have been given a whole house to ourselves; it belongs to a doctor who is on leave. This is a magnificent site, with a view over the lake nearly 10 miles to the east. The hospital is very well built and equipped.

Monday, 9 October (7:00 a.m.)

We went to bed at ten and were up shortly after six. We had a pleasant simple supper with the Buchs and Petersons—cold meat and bread and jam or cheese on one plate, with warm tea. They told us that in Denmark (they are all Danes) it is correct to rest both wrists on the table throughout the meal. They, of course, don't do this.

It is another lovely morning. Cliff and Beth Nelson were due to leave Kola Ndoto [near Shinyanga] at 5:00 a.m., so they will be on their way now. Ted has been using his tape recorder to record bird song at different places. After breakfast we will push off to meet Cliff, and will give these letters to Beth [who was to stay with Olive Burkitt]. We propose to spend tonight at Kibondo, a little over 150 miles from here.

(Later: Kigoma.) We are in a small thatched rest house. No boy has appeared. We asked the D.C. [District Commissioner] if it was booked for us, and he said yes. Cliff lit a wood fire under a big oil drum to heat our bath water and is now doing the laundry in the bathroom. Ted is cooking the supper on our primus stove. We asked in a shop if it was possible to buy either eggs or bread in this village and the answer was no. We are therefore having baked beans, biscuits, cheese, fruit, tea, and coffee.

. . . Just finished supper. Lovely meal. The tea was made in a plastic measuring jug: it was excellent. After eating the beans and bully beef on our plastic plates, Cliff produced a new roll of toilet paper to wipe the plates before putting fruit salad on them. Ted remarked, "What would Olive say?"

Beds and mattresses are provided but not bedding. We have our own. Also we have one hurricane lamp.

To go back: we met up with Cliff and Beth at 11:30 this morning, after travelling some 80 miles. They had travelled nearly 200 miles. We had a picnic lunch together and then [leaving Mrs. Nelson] we pushed on south, travelling another 100 miles through rather uninteresting bush country. It is terribly dry and dusty here. No green anywhere. Not a place one would choose to live in.

Tuesday, 10 October

(7:45 a.m.) After bath and supper last night we had a walk in the dark. There were a lot of grass fires all around. When we got back to the rest house a boy lit a pressure lamp, so we were able to read and write before going to bed. We had biscuits, bully beef, and Nescafé for breakfast.

(7:45 p.m.) We have travelled nearly 200 miles today. Yesterday we passed about one car in 10 miles. Today we passed two cars in the first 98 miles and two more in the next 70 miles. In 170 miles there was one turning off to the right and three to the left. We passed some stale elephant droppings today and yesterday but saw no game. The first 90 miles today was through endless bush. It is tsetse country and when we stopped for a few minutes to inspect the car I received several bites. They are quite harmless, but annoying.

This country is extremely thinly populated, and the people are very primitive. For the first time we saw women with masses of wire bangles around their ankles.

Kasulu was our first small township. Dirty, dusty, and altogether miserable. There was one petrol pump, but no petrol. We turned off on a diversion road up the hills to visit a Seventh Day Adventist hospital, 30 miles up through magnificent hills with the most colossal views over to Rwanda. The car boiled once, but otherwise the cooling system has been good. There have been a few minor faults. The speedometer jammed near Masaka but righted itself. A queer noise developed at Kabondo but later disappeared. The petrol tank indicator has ceased to work but this is not serious—Ted will look at it when he has time. On the whole, the car has run magnificently.

We had a picnic lunch of biscuits and beans, overlooking a superb view, and then called at the S.D.A. hospital. Very nice missionaries from South Africa, Afrikaans-speaking. I received more help with the tumour there than at any place on the trip so far. They would have loved to put us up.

The road from this hospital to Kigoma was about the most

twisty I have ever been on. Ted was driving, and went very carefully. Some sections of the road were just carved out of the side of the mountain, with a sheer drop on one side. Ted commented, "A cliff on both sides of me."

Between the Seventh Day Adventist hospital and Kigoma we descended over 3,000 feet.

Ujiji [on the eastern shore of Lake Tanganyika] is a most interesting town. Entirely African: narrow dirt streets lined with mud and wattle square houses, either thatched or covered with old flattened petrol tins, some roofed with corrugated iron. It is obviously strongly Arab, and reminds one of parts of Zanzibar.

It was almost an emotional experience visiting the Livingstone memorial, standing under the mango tree under which Livingstone and Stanley met on November 10, 1871, when my father was 15 months old. There is a great stone map of Africa with a black cross on it. Nearby is a plaque saying that Burton and Speke had visited Ujiji in 1858. We took photographs from all angles.

Kigoma is about six miles from Ujiji. We met the District Medical Officer, who directed us to the hotel and told us we must have a swim in the best pool in Africa. We followed his advice and had a lovely swim in a portion of the lake with netting around it, free from hippos and bilharzia.

The hotel is not pretentious. The bathrooms are lit by light-rays which get through a three-inch gap between the door and the lintel from a bare electric light bulb in the corridor outside. This enables you just to see the bath. Water economy is ensured by such a slow stream that few have the patience to wait for the bath to fill up with more than a couple of inches of water.

(Later: 11:00 p.m.) We had an excellent dinner with the D.M.O. We started with two empty plates plus a soup plate,

and used them one after the other as the courses arrived.
We then had two very profitable hours with the D.M.O., who
was extremely knowledgeable and gave us a great deal of
information about the tumour and all sorts of other things.

Wednesday, 11 October (8:20 p.m.)

I can't remember ever before typing by the light of a hurricane lamp—the same lamp that I bought as my first purchase
on arriving in E. Africa in the army in 1943. It is the only
lamp other than torches [flashlights] we have with us, so it
has been invaluable. We are in a rest house in the most isolated township of my experience, Mpanda.

We left Kigoma at 8:45 this morning. I have never travelled through such endless, monotonous African bush as we
did today. Mile after mile, 10 mile after 10 mile, and hundred mile after hundred mile, for 250 miles on dusty earth
roads. Everywhere was dry as dust, brown and burnt. Just
occasionally we went down an escarpment or through a pass
bordered by great rocks. On the first 60 miles to a Roman
Catholic mission we passed only one car. We were warmly
welcomed at the mission by a lady doctor and had fresh
orange drinks, and then discussed all our medical problems.
For the next 170 miles we didn't pass a single moving vehicle—just three stationary ones. We saw hardly a soul. It
really was a most desolate stretch of Africa, utterly dry and
inhospitable.

Ted was a little worried because of the occasional strange
noise in the clutch, though the engine was running magnificently. Then it began to miss, and we first thought it was
dirt in the petrol. It would stop and then start again. Finally
it stopped altogether, about 70 miles from anywhere. What
an immense comfort at such times to have a two-gallon plas-

tic bottle full of drinking water. This was Olive's Christmas present, and it has been a joy. Ted is magnificent. He nipped out of the car, and instead of spending time to find the fault he just used a piece of wire he had brought specially for the purpose, and connected the battery directly to the coil. One push of the starter, and the car went beautifully. He left the wire on until we reached Mpanda, and in twenty minutes he not only had this fault located and repaired but had repaired the petrol gauge, also an electrical fault.

We weren't sorry to reach Mpanda. While we were filling up with petrol we met the African O.C. [Officer Commanding] police, a charming chap. He found the keys of the house and led us to it. There were two bedrooms, a bathroom and water flush toilet. The other two always insist that I have the single room as leader of the expedition!

I am now writing at Sumbawanga. For supper we had two tins of spaghetti in tomato sauce, and bread and jam and tinned pears, with lots of tea. We cooked it all on our primus. A boy lit a fire under the old petrol-drum used for heating bath water and we not only bathed and shaved but I washed my hair and we even did some laundry.

After a good night, and with all the car faults fixed, we started off just after 6:00 a.m. in high spirits; and if there had been any people on the road they would have heard coming from the heavily-laden Ford the strains of hymns started by Cliff, who had brought a hymn book with music. We sang, "Will your anchor hold?", "All hail to the power," and the theme song of the Africa Inland Mission (to which both Ted and Cliff belong), "Great is thy faithfulness."

We saw some game this morning. First elephant, then kingoni, and later giraffe and sable. Ted is an honorary game ranger and can identify the animals.

Before we left Kampala we had a big metal plate fitted under our rather low petrol tank and this has been an enormous comfort. We have so often hit bottom on roads consisting of two ruts with a mound between that we would have worried about damaging our tank but for this added protection. Actually, Ted has a way of carrying on even with a holed tank, and has brought the wherewithal with him. He feeds the carburettor with a pipe direct from the petrol drum. We did once today sit on the mound of dust in the middle of the road. Cliff and I got out of the car and Ted freed it by driving backwards.

The country was much more open and interesting than it was yesterday. We passed the result of one appalling smash —a lorry literally wrapped around a tree. He must have been going too fast and left the road, and both sides of the lorry were on either side of the tree. We had to photograph it; and then took a close-up of the bumper, which had a sign, "Insure With Jubilee."

The population is sparse, and obviously very poor.

Ted is under the car; Cliff has just heated the bath water to do the laundry in the bath. Ted has now discovered the cause of the noise in the clutch. What a wonderful companion to have, or wonderful pair of companions. I couldn't wish for better. Cliff has brought a washing board and two irons!

The African houses are all square, with grass roofs. No rondavels [round huts]. We have hardly seen a bicycle between Kigoma and here, and until the last ten miles hardly a cow. What the people do for water I can't think.

Entering Sumbawanga the avenues of jacaranda were a staggering sight. The main road must have been more than half a mile long with jacaranda every ten yards on each side of the road, all a mass of blue with no green. Other avenues were the same, and in such a dry barren country it was all the more striking.

Friday, 13 October (6:16 p.m.)

(In the Abercorn Arms Hotel) I have just had a most delightful bath, the first with electric light and ample room since Bukoba. I felt I must wash my hair again, having washed it by hurricane lamp at Mpanda; but one gets quite incredibly dirty in this intensely dusty country. I also did some laundry, though Cliff accepts the laundry voluntarily.

I spent about an hour last night with the D.M.O. [District Medical Officer] and P.M.O. [Provincial Medical Officer]. We had boiled eggs for supper, and having no egg cups we gave Cliff a toilet roll, which held an egg nicely, and I used the sandwich-spread bottle, while Ted used an empty jar.

We had filled thermos flasks with tea last night, so we managed to get off just before seven this morning. The country was much more interesting—very open, with considerable hills in view. One very striking difference between this country and Uganda or Kenya is the presence of definite African villages, closely-knit bunches of houses and even sort of streets. Uganda has no villages in this sense. Moreover, all the houses are square.

We have done all our cooking on a primus stove. At meals, we take it in turn to say grace. Yesterday we passed our first thousand-mile mark, and this will have been some of our hardest travelling.

The Medical Officer [in Abercorn] is a very charming South African and a definite Christian. We discussed our business with him and he offered to take us in his Land Rover to two river falls and the southern tip of Lake Tanganyika, Mpulungu.

On our drive with him we learned a lot about the country. It is very thinly populated—only two and a half million

H

people in the vast country of Northern Rhodesia, only three million in Southern Rhodesia, and the same in Nyasaland. Yet there are 70,000 Europeans in N. Rhodesia and 350,000 in S. Rhodesia, as against 5,000 in Uganda. There are extremely few well-educated Africans, and the salaries they get are quite fantastic: over £1,000 a year for a medical assistant, not by any means equivalent to a doctor.

On the lake shore near Mpulungu we were shown the well-preserved ruin of the first mission church in this area. The London Missionary Society started work in 1883, and the church was built in 1895. This was a terrible area for trypanosomiasis [sleeping sickness], and fifteen of the first fifty missionaries died of this disease. In 1908 the whole population had to be moved 10 miles away from the lake shore.

Saturday, 14 October

(6:00 p.m. London Missionary Society Hospital, Mbereshi, near Kawambwa) We had a pleasant evening with Dr. and Mrs. van Kant yesterday. It was nice to have grace before our meal. She is a granddaughter of Dr. Robert Moffat, the well-known missionary, and has lived her life in Rhodesia. They told us many stories about the famous characters around Abercorn. One local celebrity was piloting his own plane in the London to Cairo air race in [about] 1936 and crashed at Abercorn. His companion was killed, but he married the nursing sister, who looked after him and has been there ever since.

We had breakfast at 6:30 and got away from Abercorn at seven, and then drove 250 miles through endless, interminable, identical bush, bush, BUSH, mile after mile. Most of N. Rhodesia, I believe, is like this. It had some beauty in the different shades of leaves from deep red to green, like au-

tumn tints at home. The only view is the road ahead and the
hundred yards or so that you can see between the trees. In
200 miles we passed two vehicles, a lorry and a Land Rover.
Moreover, for 230 miles there was not a single petrol pump.
Northern Rhodesia is three times the size of Uganda, with
only one third the population.

Abercorn is the place where the remnant of the German
armed forces surrendered to the British in November 1918
[at the end of World War I].

A remark I made has been frequently quoted on this
safari. From a medical point of view we must be one of the
safest safaris ever, as we are all doctors, all carry medical
supplies, and we make a bee line from one hospital to another! At breakfast yesterday we remarked that we should go
for a drive one day, just for a change!

We had a stand-up lunch of biscuits and a tin of peaches
and arrived here in time for tea. The doctor in charge here, a
Dr. Parry, worked for his first year in Africa with a Dr. P. K.
Dixon, one of the founders of the Christian union at T.C.D.
[Trinity College, Dublin].

This is a well-equipped and well-built hospital of seventy
beds. The London Missionary Society work started here at
the turn of the century. Education is, of course, a problem
for Europeans, as it is very isolated; and Mrs. Parry is at
present home with the family, leaving Dr. Parry alone for
six months. The hospital is on the Mbereshi river, which is
a tributary of the Luapala, discovered by Livingstone, and
one of the main tributaries of the Congo, near its source.

Sunday, 15 October

We went to a service in the finest mission church I have yet
been in. The segregation of the sexes is very strict, as in much

of Africa. Even the European couples sat one each side of the church. Instead of the collection being taken up, the congregation went and placed their contributions on the communion table. The service was conducted by a senior lady missionary, and she spoke to the children. The sermon was given by an African; and, of course, we understood none of it.

After service we had a cup of tea and then did a round of the hospital. It was nice to be able to help with suggestions here and there, and I am doing an operation for them at 7:15 tomorrow morning.

(Later.) We drove some six miles to a leper settlement this afternoon and were shown round by a sister who is now in Government [medical service] after thirty years in the mission. This Government settlement is run almost entirely by ex-missionaries and the head African is a local church elder.

It is actually raining, the first rain we have had since we left Uganda.

(Undated)

I last wrote on Monday morning (16 October) before leaving Mbereshi and posted the letter in Fort Rosebery. The 150-mile journey from Mbereshi was very uninteresting, just bush, bush and more bush. One gets the impression that there are hardly any people, but the roads tend to follow the watersheds to avoid bridges, while the people live in the valleys. Even so, the country is very thinly inhabited. At the turn of the century there were less than half a million people in the whole of Northern Rhodesia, which has an area at least three times that of the British Isles. There are about three million today.

We arrived at Fort Rosebery at about one o'clock. A most unattractive place, consisting of a tarmac street and a few shops, government departments, officials' houses, and a poor hotel. It is impossible to describe the utter dryness, dust and barrenness of the country at this time of the year.

We visited the hospital and discussed our business with ——, a very immature, over-confident, and incompetent young man. Some of the surgery done there is quite appalling. One good piece of fortune was that the doctor in charge of a Roman Catholic hospital some 60 miles from Fort Rosebery came in that evening, and we could discuss our problems without travelling out to her hospital. She is a doctor and a nun, with the name Mother Scholastica. I discovered she was in Trinity College, Dublin, a year behind me and knew several of the people I knew. I didn't like to ask what her name was before she entered orders.

Tuesday, 17 October

At Kasama, 224 miles from Fort Rosebery, we met two delightful doctors, Mr. Braithwaite, the P.M.O., and Dr. Wright, an ex-missionary, the D.M.O. They have a very good hospital with excellent equipment, but Dr. Wright more or less has to run the 200-bed hospital singlehanded. Braithwaite helps, but has the whole province to look after. We gained a lot of very valuable information from them, and they had seen our tumour in other places where they had worked. They asked me to look at a European lady who was in the small European hospital with abdominal pain; as Braithwaite was leaving for Ndola next morning they were worried about leaving her. I operated on her after tea, and they were very grateful. In Rhodesia they seem to have money, good equipment and good buildings, but are very short of doctors. We have infinitely more doctors but less money, poorer buildings, and worse equipment.

The road from Kasama to Abercorn runs due north. Our next stage was 120 miles due east to Tundumu, which is little more than a name on the map but has a petrol pump. We could look down into the upper end of the great Luangwa Valley. The Luangwa runs south for some 600 miles to join the Zambesi at Zomba and only one road crosses it near its southern end. Livingstone had to return his porters to the country near Zomba, after he brought them on his journey across Africa and back to Tete. Yesterday I was reading the description of this journey, which he made with Dr. Kirk in 1858. I never before appreciated the difficulty of trekking on foot through country like this.

We passed our 2,000-mile mark between Abercorn and Tundumu. A few miles before Tundumu we turned off to a small hospital which was formerly run by the mission but is now staffed by Government [medical personnel]. The doctor in charge is a well-known personality—a very wide-awake lady of over eighty, Dr. Trant, who trained at Trinity College, Dublin. She was able to give us information about one case of the tumour we are investigating, which came from the upper part of the Luangwa Valley—very valuable information.

The road improved after Tundumu, running southeast to Nyasaland, which has been called the Switzerland of Africa. We were aiming for a rest house which we knew to be situated in a most impressive setting. We hadn't booked it, and hoped it would be available. In all we covered some 320 miles and arrived here shortly after four o'clock and, fortunately, it was empty. The view is quite superb, with magnificent mountains about four miles away.

It is incredible how much dust you pick up on a trip like

this one. Everything gets impregnated with dust. I washed shirts, vests, stockings, etc., before my bath last night, and had to change the brown water repeatedly. I then washed my hair in the bath water before bathing, and immediately the water was thick brown. One really feels a bath is worthwhile!

For supper we had two fried eggs each with nearly a pound of bacon between us, and baked beans. Then a tin of pineapple, and tea. Our butter has turned to oil floating on top of a white sediment, something I have never seen before.

Saturday, 21 October (5:45 a.m.)

I am at Livingstonia, overlooking perhaps the finest view in the Federation. This is the famous Church of Scotland mission station perched more than 2,000 feet above Lake Nyasa.

The journey from Karonga to Livingstonia yesterday was most interesting. The first 30 miles is through country with numerous palms and baobab trees (which look like trees uprooted and then planted upside down with the roots in the air). Next, some 30 miles of bush. Then we turned to the mountains and climbed the most colossal, terrific and almost terrifying mountain road I have ever been up. We thought the road from Lake Thun to Beattenburg was steep and twisty, but it was just a slightly curved road with an occasional gradient compared to this. I have never, ever, anywhere, been on such a road. It climbed over 2,000 feet in seven miles, which was only about two miles as the crow flies. There were 112 bends and 22 hairpin turns doubling back virtually 180°. Moreover, at these hairpin bends the turn was so steep that our car could only just make it in bottom gear. On six of the bends we just couldn't get round in one turn even with the wheels fully locked, and had to back on the corner. Fortunately, the corners are constructed to make this possible or one couldn't get up at all. The radiator boiled repeatedly and we had to refill it and pour water over it to help the cooling.

When we reached the top we certainly had our reward, in perhaps the finest view in the Federation. We are staying with the doctor and his wife. Dr. Maclean was in the past Deputy Director of Medical Services in Tanganyika, then Director in Trinidad. After retiring from Government he came out as a missionary with the U.M.C.S. He then retired again, but after hearing an appeal for a doctor to come out here, he returned. He is now seventy-two, and one admires him enormously. We were given an empty room and a balcony overlooking the lake. We put up our camp beds with our own bedding. Mrs. Maclean is seventy-nine, and what a remarkable character! Bubbling over with humour, and such a lady. The two of them are just like a Victorian couple from a very refined family stuck in the middle of Africa. Their manner, and all about them, is cultured and radiant with Christian sweetness. In this old rambling house, so much in need of repair, there was a silver tea-pot, and nice china, and good table linen.

Monday, 23 October

We went to morning service yesterday at Ekwendeni, in a large red brick church. We were impressed by the very poor quality of dress. A man who was leading the community singing before the service started was dressed much more shabbily than our garden boy on Sunday. As in nearly all African churches there was a strict segregation of the sexes, men on one side and women on the other.

Dr. Ken Irvine runs the hospital with no medical help.

At present he has no [nursing] sister. This means that he never really gets off, and he has all the buildings and engines and electrical fittings to look after, as well as patients. I do admire enormously the sacrifices such a man is prepared to make, not the least being the professional isolation. Another sacrifice is the primitive latrine, a tin hut in the yard with a box over a deep pit.

It's very hot, as hot as we ever get it in Kampala, but cooler at night. Ken has the same text on his wall as we had seen at the outset of our safari on the wall of the Indian D.M.O.'s house at Bukoba: "Christ is the head of this house, the unseen guest at every meal, the silent listener to every conversation."

He has a girl, instead of a boy, to help in the house, and she served our supper with a baby, fast asleep, strapped to her back!

We were up at five this morning and off at six. Cliff remarked that an unusual aspect of this safari is that we always seem to start *before* the time scheduled! We drove, first, east to Mzuzu, the Provincial Headquarters, and then south over the very lovely Vipya plateau—some 50 miles of the most delightful country. There seemed to be virtually no population, but good areas of afforestation, and large plantations of *tung* which they are growing for the useful oil.

Mzimba is some 80 miles from Ekwendeni. We met the African doctor, a Nyasa man who spent seventeen years in South Africa and was at Fort Hare and Witwatersrand in Johannesburg. Unfortunately, they no longer admit [black] Africans there. Bwanausi is his name; he had only recently come to Mzimba but had served in Port Herald, in the extreme south of the country, where he had seen five of the tumours in seven months. We must visit this hospital.

Ken Irvine had given us a letter to leave with a mission-

H*

ary on the outskirts of Mzimba. We met a charming couple who were obviously radiant Christians. We asked where they came from, and they replied, a place called Enniskillen in N. Ireland! We found then that we had many mutual friends, and they asked if I was a son of J. P. Burkitt! Such an unexpected and pleasant contact in the middle of Africa.

It was about 170 miles from Mzimba to Fort Jamieson, where I am writing. The country is similar to the rest of Northern Rhodesia, though I was impressed by the lovely green and brown fresh new leaves coming up in virtual desert earth. The strange thing is that all these fresh green shoots come out *before* the rain, and *in anticipation of it.* Really quite remarkable.

"What unusual methods of doing research," we remarked, "and how pleasant." One usually associated research with white coats and test tubes.

We arrived at Fort Jamieson at four and went to the hospital. I met a sister, and asked if I could ring up the P.M.O. I told him I was looking into some children's jaw tumours. The sister, overhearing this, sent to the ward and produced an absolutely typical case of the tumour we have been looking for. I have been back since to photograph it and take notes. This is very important for our work.

I have just had a bath and hair wash. One really does enjoy them on this trip. Cliff is an absolute brick, and has just been round for my laundry. Ted has been under the car, making sure all is well. I couldn't have had two more congenial colleagues. Ted has a very great knowledge of medicine and was obviously an unusually good student. Cliff, too, is obviously a very good and dedicated brain. Although I am leader of the party I feel in many ways intellectually behind them, but have had more opportunities.

Tuesday, 24 October

It is 90 miles from Fort Jamieson to Lilongwe. Uninteresting
bush. For part of the way the road runs along the border between Rhodesia and Mozambique. We reached here about
2:30 and spent some time in the hospital. A sister showed us
round one of the wards, and I asked where she came from.
She replied that she came from a town in N. Ireland called
Enniskillen! Fancy meeting two—no, three—people from Enniskillen in the heart of Africa in two days. Her name is
Sherriden.

Ted is making all the entries in the cash-book. He does
this most professionally and meticulously, and it saves me a
lot of work. I leave all the finance to him, and just draw the
money from the bank.

Friday, 27 October

(Blantyre) We had dinner last night with Mr. Laycock (the
surgeon at the hospital here) and his wife. He has had a very
wide experience, having served in China, Somaliland, Tanganyika, and Nyasaland. He and his wife married in Somaliland seven weeks after first meeting. At the birth of their
child a doctor was to fly from Aden. At the last moment he
couldn't come, and Laycock eventually had to do a Caesarean
section on his own wife, assisted only by Somali orderlies.
His wife was a tutor sister, and she sat up on the trolley in
the [operating] theatre and checked the instruments before
she was given the anaesthetic!

This morning I did a thyroidectomy on invitation, and
then we went and visited the Director and his deputy. This
is always a diplomatic move. They showed great interest in
our work and offered every assistance.

Monday, 30 October

(Beira) We all slept well, but were up by 5:30, and spent most of the morning at the hospital trying to describe our tumour to Portuguese doctors who knew some English. Quite a strain. Eventually one who had worked in America joined us and helped with interpretation. Quite obviously the tumour is common throughout this country, as we had anticipated. They actually produced one classical case for us.

We have been asked to have drinks with some of the senior members of the staff. I hope there is some light wine that we can get down without too much difficulty. After that we propose to try a Chinese restaurant for supper.

Tuesday, 31 October

(Umtali) We are in a new world. After weeks of heat and dust and drought it has rained in a continual drizzle all day, just like the United Kingdom, and we have been cool again. Last night we went round to the house of the Beira surgeon. A beautiful house, with exquisite furniture imported from Lisbon and Macao, off the China coast. It was air-conditioned, and no money had been spared on it. The daughters, aged about twelve and fourteen, came in, and the younger kissed us all. We struggled through a glass of port wine and ate nuts and cake.

The shops are well stocked with beautiful things, all imported. There is no doubt that the Portuguese have built a magnificent modern town at Beira. The architectural styles, with bizarre colours and totally unorthodox shapes, were really exciting and often very pleasing.

We left Beira before eight this morning in the rain, and enjoyed the 186 miles of tarmac road through green country, with mists hanging over the hills as in Scotland. It was most interesting to us to find that the first hospital we visited, at 2,000 feet, was obviously above the belt where the tumours occur. This was further evidence to confirm our theory.

Umtali is a quite magnificent town. We seem to have returned to civilization completely in the past two days. There are masses of flowering shrubs, various shades of bougain-villaea, carpets of fallen blue petals under the jacaranda trees, well-kept parks and trim lawns. It is all so obviously a European town. Magnificent shops, where you are served by English men and women. It is smaller than Nairobi but much more attractive.

First impressions of the hospital are also very favourable. We are looking around tomorrow, and I am giving a lecture tomorrow evening.

We have decided to be gay tonight, and to go to the cinema to see the life of Franz Liszt.

I imagine colour segregation is pretty acute here, and the cinema is for Europeans only. We have never come across this before.

(Wednesday evening)

We had dinner at the club with Dr. Montgomery. He told us there was at least one Enniskillen man in Umtali, a name not known to me.

Friday, 3 November

(Salisbury) Yesterday's drive was by far the most beautiful of our whole trip. We LONGED to have our wives with us. We left Umtali shortly after 7:30 and drove to Salisbury via Inyanga, marvelously beautiful mountain scenery. The road, the scenery, and the weather, were all superb. Great rocky hills, immense vistas, patterns of wattle plantations, and Paul Henry clouds. Changing views all the time and crisp fresh air. The hilltops were wrapped with flimsy mantles of drifting cloud. I have never seen so many examples of rocks and great smooth boulders perched precariously on top of one another. For mile after mile we were entranced by these queer bundles of enormous stones, many apparently about to topple over. I suppose this is due to rain and wind, over the centuries, removing the supporting earth.

We reached Salisbury at about 4:00 p.m. The approach is very like Nairobi, with pleasant houses and well laid-out gardens, and masses of bougainvillaea and jacaranda. As one approaches the town it is like suddenly striking Manhattan in the middle of Africa. Quite a remarkable sight: a skyline of skyscrapers.

Saturday, 4 November

After breakfast yesterday Mr. Hammer, one of the local surgeons, drove us around Salisbury. A very fine city indeed. We spent most of the morning in the hospital and met many of the staff. A magnificent and well-equipped institution. There is so much more money here than in E. Africa, and of course a considerable number of private surgeons and physicians and specialists.

We had lunch with the radiologist. The house seemed entirely furnished with delicate antique furniture, Louis XV chairs with tapered legs and covered with tapestry. The cupboards were filled with Dresden and other china, and cut glass was strewn about in profusion. I must say that I would long for a comfortable chair or sofa I could relax in.

After lunch I had an appointment with the Director of Medical Services. There had been an absurd farce arising from our visit. I had written to one of his deputies months ago announcing my coming. This was just for courtesy and required no action. The deputy, however, was a stickler for red tape, and referred the matter to Rhodesia House in London. Not knowing what to do, they referred it to the Colonial Office. They, in turn, contacted the Imperial Cancer Research Fund and other bodies. Even the Prime Minister here was asked if he knew about my coming! All utter rubbish. I have now cleared up any misunderstanding. I don't know what they thought I was going to do to the Federation.

Sunday, 5 November

Ted and I very much enjoyed a very nice service in a Methodist church. It was strange to us to see a cross in a Methodist church.

After service we visited the hospital to find the doctor. He was not in, but a sister from Newry, Co. Down, gave us a cup of tea and put us on the phone to Dr. Stover. Later he came round to our hotel, and we had a long talk and derived much information from his continuous twenty-five years here. There are a number of doctors in S. Rhodesian towns who have refused promotion and who might have been Directors by now but preferred to remain in one place and make it their home. Dr. Montgomery has been twenty-five years in Umtali, and a Dr. MacGladdery (another Irishman) has been twenty-five years at Owelo. A Dr. ———, also of Irish descent, has lived for thirty-five years in a small town some distance from here.

After lunch we drove out to the famous Zimbabwe ruins, probably the most famous and mysterious archaeological remains in all Africa. A quite fantastic sight. There is one structure, called the temple, some 50 yards across, with great walls of cut stone 40 feet high and some 4 to 6 feet thick. Within this huge circular wall there are the remains of many buildings, and scattered for many acres around it are other buildings in poor preservation. Then, on a neighbouring hill covered with enormous rock boulders there are steps, and remains of buildings which make use of the boulders as walls and arches, so that the whole thing is like an uncovered rabbit warren with paths running in and out of the rocks, and often under them. These ruins have been dated back to between the eighth and twelfth centuries A.D., using methods employing measurement of radioactivity. The remarkable thing is that a civilization existed, capable of building structures of this nature; and then for a thousand years nothing more elaborate than mud huts were built. It would seem that a whole civilization disappeared, rather as happened on Easter Island in the Pacific.

Later we drove out to see Dr. —— referred to above. We felt we must draw on his long experience of nearly thirty-five years in one station. We found his lonely house; and he was having a typical bachelor tea. He was a stout man, not looking his sixty-three years, but when we talked to him his brain was that of an older man and he had difficulty collecting his thoughts. The reason was, I think, long years of excessive whiskey and gin. He wasn't really able to help us very much, and we realized that he found memory and concentration difficult. He had been a great hunter in his time, and had actually shot over 800 buffalo. Not many men have done this. The guest room was rather unusually furnished, 49 framed pictures, nearly all of dead game, with a few African gun bearers, and one bottle of scent together with some talcum powder! He also had framed on the walls of another room some photographs of larger tumours and other medical conditions he had seen. We felt very sorry for him. Obviously a thoroughly unhappy and disillusioned man. We noticed that he was reading some religious books, and we thought we might post him something that might be helpful.

Wednesday, 8 November

(Pretorius Kop camp, at lower end of Kruger National Park) We have just returned from seven hours in the park, and had a wonderful time. We must have seen a thousand impala in all. We also saw lots of wart hogs, water buck, gnu, kadu, one elephant, one sable antelope (a very large animal). We had some remarkable experiences. I was about to photograph some vervet monkeys when one with a baby on her breast jumped up and actually sat with her baby on the ledge of the car window at my shoulder. It was too close to photograph! Later we encountered some baboons, usually shy animals. As I was getting ready to photograph them one jumped in the open window and sat on the back of the seat behind my neck! Ted had to chase it out.

Friday, 10 November

We were up at five yesterday morning and left the park at about 6:45. It was a very pleasant and easy drive to Lourenço Marques. We chose a hotel from a guide book; very comfortable, central, and not expensive.

After a light lunch we went to the hospital to make contact with a Prof. Prates, the best-known name in medicine in Mozambique. I had been in correspondence with him. He welcomed us cordially and showed us the work he has been doing. We saw his records and some lovely plaster models of patients with tumours and other lesions, made by a man who worked at the museum but who is now dead. We recognized

our own particular tumour among these models. In his office
we met the representative of a drug firm from Johannesburg,
a Mr. Thomas, and later in the evening he very kindly gave
us supper in one of the cafes.

I should mention that the sisters in the hospital are, of
course, nuns, and they seem extremely good. The white bed-
linen would completely shame Mulago Hospital.

The above was written after lunch. It is now 6:30, Friday
evening, and it has been an extraordinarily interesting day.

We had breakfast in the hotel at 7 and then all three of
us went down town and decided to have a haircut. It was a
real experience. While my hair was being cut a boy gave my
shoes a superb polish, making them look like new. A lady
with highly painted and polished nails wanted to manicure
mine, but I declined. The haircut took as long as a major
operation, and included being smothered in talcum powder,
drenched in sprayed scent, and drowned in hair oil. Even
my eyebrows were trimmed. All this cost me more than 6/-,
but the three of us walked out of the shop feeling real
dandies. The whole car was fragrant with perfume. It was a
particularly novel experience for Ted as his hair is usually
cut by Muriel, and he hasn't been to a barber for years.

After this we went to the hospital and had the most useful morning of our whole trip. Prates has his records beautifully tabulated and we were able to get out the records of all
children's cancers for the past five years. We made notes on
over forty cases of the tumour we are investigating and also
got their addresses so that we can plot them on a map. As
Lourenço Marques is the most southerly place from which
the tumour has been reported this information is of very great
value. We also took photographs of the magnificent models
he has collected, and these will add real spice to lectures
when used as illustrations. Not only did we get this valuable

information on lymphomas, but we also got valuable information on other tumours. Prates is certainly a remarkable
man and his records must be almost unique.

Sunday, 12 November

(Mount Hermon Mission, Mankaiana, Swaziland South African General Mission) Supper with Prof. Prates and Mr.
Thomas, the drug firm representative, on Friday night in
Lourenço Marques, was another experience. Prates took us
to a cafe, where he seemed to know everyone. After selecting
a table he disappeared, in order to inspect the prawns prior
to cooking! We had the special Mozambique dish of enormous
prawns, like little lobsters, grilled and served in rather strong
sauce. They were very delicious. Bread is provided in the
form of long loaves which are cut in two. Each person helps
himself to half a loaf, which is lovely and fresh. We three
drank Coca-Cola and tried some light wine, but I found it
ghastly stuff. Prates and Thomas got through quite a lot of
whiskey.

Prates is really a great character. Definitely the personality of the medical world in Mozambique, and very excellent
at his job. He has done quite remarkable work with very
limited staff and facilities. You can understand that he
doesn't like being treated as a "dago" by some young white
South African, and he was telling us of occasions when he
was over-exasperated and just jumped over the counter at
some office or airport to smack the fellow on the face or report him to the government.

(Swaziland) We called at a large and very fine hospital
run by "The Church of the Nazarene," very fine Christian
people. This is at Manzini. There are three doctors at this
hospital, and they have 250 beds, a great number for a mis-

sion hospital. The senior doctor insisted that we stay for lunch, and we found him and his wife very charming: his father was one of the medical pioneers out here, while she comes from London. The buildings are some of the finest we have ever seen at any mission hospital. It was a very useful contact for us from a scientific standpoint as they do not see the tumour we are hunting, and their long experience is a more valuable "negative" than a "no" from a government doctor with only a few years' experience.

Tuesday, 14 November

(Johannesburg) Morning service in the little church at Mankaiana was—as in most African churches—with all the men on one side and all the women on the other. It was characterized by a sermon lasting about 50 minutes, which tends to be tedious when in an unknown language. In contrast to Uganda, the married women all had some covering on their heads.

Cliff spoke to a boys' Bible class in the afternoon, and I spoke at a weekly prayer-meeting in the evening. We had agreed that if we were invited to speak we would take it in turn. Ted had his first turn at Mbereshi.

We left Mankaiana at 6:45 yesterday, and the 260-mile drive to Johannesburg was most interesting. Swaziland is a very attractive country: there is no dividing line between it and Eastern Transvaal—it continues as vast rolling hills covered with short green grass and patterned with wattle plantations and attractive bungalow farmsteads, like an enormous version of the Sussex Downs. This vast, open, arable country stretches for over a hundred miles.

We saw many instances of teams of oxen ploughing—the old methods persist alongside the modern. In fact, we passed one old couple with bowed heads sitting in a trap drawn by two donkeys, proceeding along the road at about one and a half miles an hour, a striking contrast to the great American cars dashing past. I suppose the old Boer trekkers covered hundreds of miles at this snail's pace.

After we got to Springs, some 30 miles east of Johannesburg, we were virtually in built-up territory for the rest of our journey. Such a contrast to what we have seen of Africa on this trip, with miles and miles of nothing and stretches of a hundred miles with hardly another vehicle on the road. We might almost have been approaching Birmingham—a succession of towns, and in every direction the great man-made mountains of soil turned up by innumerable mines. Some of these are like great pyramids, others just truncated pyramids with bases several hundred yards long, but still growing. The traffic was reminiscent of English roads, with streams of great heavy lorries. Fortunately, we had a map to help us to find our way through the maze of streets and skyscrapers to the South African Institute for Medical Research. There we met Dr. Oettlé, who is arranging our programme. We found a great and welcome mail waiting for us, and after some preliminary discussions we were directed to a hotel into which we'd been booked. A *much* more pretentious hotel than we would ever have chosen for ourselves, each in a single room with private bath.

My lecture to the Institute staff was scheduled for 5:10. It was very well attended and extremely well received, almost embarrassingly so. The discussion that followed gave me a great deal of information which was most helpful. They have now found two cases of this tumour in South Africa, where it was believed to be unknown.

We were brought out to dinner with Mr. Thomas, the drug firm representative we met in Lourenço Marques, to-

gether with his wife and an American scientist who works for
the same company in a research capacity. We went to one of
those restaurants which it is an experience to visit occasionally if the meal is being charged on someone else's expense
account: carpeted floors, subdued lights, waiters in dress
suits, and everything on the menu three times the price it
would be elsewhere.

After dinner we were brought to the hotel where the
American is staying (rather more pretentious than our hotel)
and we got down to shop. Ted and Cliff are going to do some
trials on a new drug for schistosomiasis [bilharzia], which is
common in the areas where they work. I promised I would
ask one of our physicians to do the same. If they can get
their drug pushed it is worth spending £6 on dinner. But I
must emphasize that Thomas has been most helpful, and I
believe he brought us out for kindness.

Wednesday, 15 November

Our first session yesterday was with a pathologist who had
seen a European child with the tumour syndrome we are investigating. This will be the first time it has been described
in a European. Although the child lives here, it had been to
lower altitudes for holidays, a significant fact.

We were then brought to the great Baragwanath African
hospital standing near the enormous "Native locations" south
of the city. This is the largest hospital in the southern hemisphere. The traffic on our way out was terrific—three and four
lanes all going the same way. I believe there is one car for
every three people in Johannesburg. It is a hutted type of
hospital, covering therefore a very large area. Excellent work
seems to be done there and the staff are really keen. We were
very warmly welcomed and shown different departments and

wards by various members of the staff. . . . We got the impression that a large section of the whites, including many of the staff of the Baragwanath, don't favour the [racial] policy of the present government.

We all picked up many useful tips in this hospital to bring back to our respective units. Ted is always on the lookout for what he can adopt for Kuluva, and I think it is wonderful what he manages to do there.

Thursday, 16 November

Yesterday was, if anything, an even more full and interesting day than Tuesday. We were first driven out to the Virus Research Unit, about 7 miles from here. A full programme was laid on for us so that we could meet the workers in charge of the various departments. We saw tissue cultures of living cells and the maps of distribution of various viruses. Whatever virus is responsible for our tumour, and whatever insect carries it, must of course exist in the specific areas where the tumour occurs. We were given all sorts of interesting lines of thought to follow up.

We spent the afternoon at the Institute for Medical Research with the expert on maps, distribution of insects, animals and vegetation, etc. This was relevant to our problem—to find out what factors may be responsible for the distribution of the tumour. We were able to procure a lot of useful maps to bring back to Kampala.

(Later) Oettlé brought us out to his home, four miles out in the suburbs. We went by double-decker bus, and Ted particularly enjoyed it as he hasn't done any "strap-hanging" for many years.

We found George Oettlé and his wife a delightful Christian couple. Plymouth Brethren. They have six children under the age of nine, the youngest being two weeks. We all sat around a big table, and George gave thanks. Then, after the meal, before the children went to bed, they all gathered round and each in turn read a couple of verses of the chapter of Scripture for the day. Then George led us all as we knelt in prayer. It was such a very pleasant, free, happy evening. Oettlé is a world name in cancer research, and last year he was at conferences in Tokyo, England, Kampala, etc. Next year he is due in Moscow, Philadelphia, Dakar, and other places. This travelling is, of course, most interesting, but he and his wife hate parting. As I said before, we three have found that the only cloud over this trip.

This morning we are due to meet three more authorities in different subjects, and then we have lunch with the Professor of Surgery before spending the afternoon with Prof. Murray and Oettlé. We shall feel quite exhausted when we leave here, but it has been enormously valuable. We leave Johannesburg early tomorrow for Pietersburg. We are due to spend this evening again with the Oettlés.

That evening, after supper with the children and family prayers, an elderly lady of eighty who was staying with the Oettlés played the piano "beautifully," and Mrs. Oettlé ("who," Burkitt remarks, "has a very fine trained voice") sang several solos accompanied by her friend. Ted Williams also played the piano, and so did one of the children ("a nine-year-old daughter, who plays extraordinarily well").

This marked the end of the first half of the safari. The following morning, Friday, 17 November, at 8:30, the three men left Johannesburg on the return trip to Kampala. They encountered tremendous rainstorms as they approached Uganda, the worst seen in a hundred years; again and again

*the stationwagon had to be dug out of the mud; and on one
stretch of road it took them nearly three and a half hours to
cover fifteen miles. On Sunday, 17 December, they arrived at
Mulago, and the final entry in the* Lymphoma Safari Diary
describes the homecoming.

Sunday, 17 December

(Mulago) We left Mbale at 6:30 on Thursday morning and
reached the road block beyond Tororo at about 7:30. There
was a row of lorries in front of us and a police post at either
end of a quarter of mile of road over which water was flowing pretty rapidly. It was just possible for vehicles to get
through in single-line traffic, one way at a time. The water
was up to the floor boards of the car and the road very rough,
but we got through. There was one bus upside down in the
swamp at one side of the road, with its wheels and part of
the chassis above the level of the water. There were two lorries on their sides, and one Land Rover in the swamp. Several people had been drowned here the previous day. After
getting through I took off my shoes and stockings and waded
half way back to take photographs of cars getting through
and of the vehicles in the swamp.

At Bugiri we telephoned Olive to announce our arrival at
Mulago about noon. We stopped for a little at Jinja to photograph the unusual gush of water coming through the sluice
gates at the Jinja dam. When we reached Mulago at 12:10
we found palm leaves along each side of the entrance to our
house laced with colored bunting, and a "Welcome Home"
arch. We were showered with confetti from the families, all
three wives being there to meet us, and Molly Williams,
Judy and Rachel and Geoffrey Nelson. After the greeting,

Ted took the car out again to get photographs of it coming home! And thus happily ended the safari of a lifetime.

And yesterday, Ted was backing the car just outside the house and went too near a slippery bank, and got badly stuck in the mud. We had to dig him out!

Our hearts are full of thankfulness to God for all His mercies to us.

The trip is over, the diary closes. I hope you have found it of some interest.

Our love to you all.